The Traveling Woman

The Traveling Woman

Great Tips for Safe and Healthy Trips

Catherine Comer
and
Lavon Swaim

IMPACT PUBLICATIONS
Manassas Park, Virginia

The Traveling Woman

Library of Congress Cataloging-in-Publication Data

Comer, Catherine
 The traveling woman: great tips for safe and healthy trips /
  Catherine Comer, Lavone Swaim
   p. cm.—
 Includes bibliographical references
 ISBN 1-57023-161-3
 1. Travel. 2. Women Travelers. I. Swaim, Lavon. II. Title.

G151.C66 2001
910'.2'02—dc   2001024171

Publisher: For information on Impact Publications, including current and forthcoming publications, authors, press kits, bookstore, and submission requirements, visit Impact's Web site: *www.impactpublications.com.*

Publicity-Rights: For information on publicity, author interviews, and subsidiary rights, contact the Media Relations Department: Tel. 703-361-7300 Fax 703-335-9486 or email *travel@impactpublications.com.*

Sales-Distribution: All bookstore sales are handled through Impact's trade distributor: National Book Network, 15200 NBN Way, Blue Ridge Summit, PA 17214, Tel. 1-800-462-6420. All other sales and distribution inquiries should be directed to the publisher: Sales Department, IMPACT PUBLICATIONS, 9104 Manassas Drive, Suite N, Manassas Park, VA 20111-5211, Tel. 703-361-7300, Fax 703-335-9486, or email: *sales@impactpublications.com.*

Book design by Kristina Ackley; Layout by Stacy Noyes

Contents

Acknowledgments

We gratefully acknowledge the following individuals and companies for their support and assistance.

Don Comer & Ken Swaim

Stephen Grubowski

U.S. State Department

U.S. Customs Service

Rochelle Sobel, Association for Safe International
Road Travel

Travel Industry Association of America

U.S. Department of Transportation

Ricki Pollycove, MD, MHS

Consul General Larry Colbert & Staff, U.S.
Consulate, Paris

Sergeant Michael Janin, City of Beaverton Police
  Department

Leonard & Anne Grubowski

Mary Catherine Tubbs

Shirley Reeves

Louise Brett

Patricia Mounier, Louvre Museum, Paris

American Express

U.S. Bank Visa

Richard Ransome

Monique Bond

Jim Boehner

Ruby Edwards

Ray Flynt, Travelers Aid International

Tayee, Blue Planet Hostel

Carol Rossman, U.S. Bank

Shaun Hughes, Sun Precautions, Inc.

Ron and Caryl Krannich

Mardie Younglof

Thank you to our families and friends for their love, support, and encouragement.

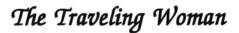

The Traveling Woman

Introduction

Do you dream of a gentle sea breeze drifting over your face as you gaze into the deep, blue Mediterranean; or your first glimpse of the Eiffel Tower aglow in the Paris night? Or maybe you fantasize about climbing the Great Wall of China, trekking through the Australian Outback, or sailing through a shopping spree at exotic ports of call? Maybe you are a businesswoman who travels on your job or a student planning to study abroad. The world holds incredible discoveries for women to experience, regardless of their age and whether traveling for business or leisure.

As we lingered over a glass of wine on a warm spring evening in San Antonio, Texas, we pondered the many destinations throughout the world we have yet to discover and dreamed of where we might travel next. We lived in two different parts of the United States and had decided to meet in San Antonio for four days of relaxation and catching up.

We were reviewing our packing list for an upcoming trip to Europe and daydreaming about the exciting places we would

1

visit, when we were abruptly brought "down to earth" with a news report of two women travelers who had been attacked while in a taxi in Mexico. As we discussed this tragedy, we thought of how we could keep ourselves safe as we traveled. The news did not diminish our desire to travel but, rather, sparked our motivation to find out how to travel with safety in mind. We wondered how many women do not experience the delights of travel because of *fear*: it could be fear of being a crime victim while traveling, becoming ill while away from home, or simply being afraid of the unknown in a foreign country. These are serious concerns for today's traveling woman.

We began to recall our travel experiences. As two women who have been traveling for the last 20 years, we thought about problems we had encountered while on our trips.

"Remember the time," Catherine said, "when my luggage did not make it to Madrid and how frightened I was to be left alone in a hotel room in a foreign country where I spoke only a little of the language? And when my credit card was canceled while I was touring England?" "Oh yes," Lavon added, "and remember when I had to sleep on the floor of the Cordoba Airport in Argentina when our flight was delayed and there were armed guards roaming throughout the terminal? I was not prepared for that sight!" "And," Catherine winced, "when we lost one of our traveling ladies on the subway in Seoul?"

As we reviewed travel plans that had gone awry, we continued to share stories ranging from small inconveniences to incidents when we were placed in danger. We talked of trips when we suffered from ailments such as traveler's diarrhea, and confessed to unwise decisions such as when we opted to take the subway late at night in Paris. Instead of having the restaurant staff call a taxi, we chose to ride the subway and found ourselves on a dark deserted street, looking for the entrance to the station.

We thought of things we could have done differently to protect ourselves and stay healthy while traveling, and we wondered how many women travelers have these same concerns. We wondered if women travel differently than men, and if so, how?

We decided to research travel safety and health for women and gather information to share with women of all ages the importance of keeping these issues in mind when traveling.

Our endeavor began in Washington, D.C., at the U.S. State Department. We met with a State Department representative to find out what types of problems U.S. citizens experience when traveling. We learned that most incidents occur because travelers are not properly prepared while traveling. Problems such as stolen money and passports are common because many travelers are not aware of how to carry valuables safely. We were also told that sometimes people put themselves at risk because they do not know enough about the area in which they are traveling. This can be critical if they are in countries for which travel advisories have been posted.

At the U.S. Customs headquarters, seasoned agents explained how to make the Customs process easier. Our concern for travel safety was validated again with our trip to the U.S. Department of Transportation, where we learned that their studies on women's travel issues report that women do care about travel safety. We met with the founder of the Association for Safe International Road Travel who shared the tragic story of how her son was killed while traveling on a bus in Turkey.

Approximately 60 million U.S. residents travel by air to foreign destinations annually and millions more travel domestically.

With female adults representing about 40 percent of these travelers, we knew we were on the right track in our concern for women's travel safety and health. Women face unique issues while traveling, ranging from health issues such as yeast and bladder infections to safety concerns such as how to protect ourselves physically from purse snatchers or muggers. We discovered that many American women unknowingly place themselves in precarious situations because of our nature of being outgoing and friendly. We may not realize that in many foreign countries this can be an invitation for unwanted male advances, or can even signal criminals that we are obviously tourists and may be carrying large sums of money. Along the way, we learned many travel tips to share with you, such as how to pack lightly without straining your back with a 50-pound carry-on, and how handy a small flashlight can be in an emergency.

To bring you this edition of *The Traveling Woman, Great Tips for Safe and Healthy Trips,* we have interviewed experienced travel planners, security professionals, Customs agents, doctors specializing in women's travel needs, and national and international authorities on travel safety. We discovered how to consider health and safety issues while in the trip-planning stages, how to deal with a variety of health issues, and even tips for staying in touch with loved ones at home. Our passion is for traveling and our hope is that you can fulfill your travel dreams safely. We invite you to follow these tips chapter by chapter. Plan carefully, act wisely, take precautions, and most of all...

Enjoy a safe and healthy trip!!

Before you begin your journey, take our test on page 5 to see how savvy you are when it comes to travel health and safety issues.

What's Your Travel Health and Safety IQ?

Today's traveling woman has many opportunities to enjoy travel to destinations around the world. However, we believe that an educated traveler is a safer traveler and arming ourselves with knowledge on how to protect our belongings and ourselves while traveling will help insure a more enjoyable travel experience.

Test your travel health and safety IQ with this quick quiz by answering yes or no to the following questions. Add up your points to see how ready you are for your next trip. Good luck.

1. I always research my destination before traveling to find ways to stay safe and healthy while on my trip.

    Yes 5   No 0

2. When making a hotel reservation, I always ask for a room on the second floor near the elevator because this is considered a safer location than the first floor or rooms near exterior exits.

    Yes 5   No 0

3. I have a copy of my health insurance policy in my travel file and know what is covered while I am traveling both domestically and internationally.

    Yes 5   No 0

4. When traveling on an airplane, I flex my feet and point my toes every two hours to increase circulation.

    Yes 5   No 0

5. When entering an elevator, I stand near the controls with my back against the wall so that I have access to floor buttons and the emergency alarm while being able to view anyone coming or going.

    Yes 5   No 0

6. If my passport is lost or stolen while traveling, I know to call the police first to obtain a police report for the consulate replacement procedures.

Yes 5   No 0

7. I avoid being a potential target for criminals by carrying valuables in a hidden money belt.

Yes 5   No 0

8. I always access the U.S. State Department website before traveling to foreign countries to receive a country profile and find out about any travel advisories that may be posted.

Yes 5   No 0

9. I always pack a small first aid kit while traveling and include adhesive bandages, ointments such as anti-itching, antibiotic, and insect repellent, diarrhea medication, sun protection lotion, antacid pills, and anti-bacterial towelettes.

Yes 5   No 0

10. When renting a car in a foreign country, I apply for an International Driver's Permit before leaving.

Yes 5   No 0

Total score _____

If you scored a perfect 50, congratulations on being a savvy traveler. If you answered no to any of these questions, you may be placing yourself in a vulnerable position while traveling. You may not be aware of potential problems and how to deal with them. Read on to discover great resources to assist you in your travel planning, and tips to help you protect yourself while on the road, in the air, or out to sea. Our goal is for you to become a safe and healthy traveling woman!

1

Researching Your Destination

Whether traveling around the state or around the world, researching your destination can be an exciting part of your trip. Make this fun! Grab your favorite cup of coffee, relax and enjoy discovering your travel destination. Whether you use an agent, the Internet, or call yourself to book your travel, make it a priority to find out as much as you can about the area and what there is to see and do while you are there. Knowing you have planned well can help ease the stress that sometimes accompanies travel, especially when traveling internationally. As you plan your trip, begin to think of ways to keep yourself and your belongings safe. Soon, you can make this part of your lifestyle, just as locking doors has become a habit for most women when they get in the car. Practicing good safety habits can help you enjoy your destination.

Planning wisely will not only help ensure a safer travel experience, it will also enable you to be flexible with your itinerary once you arrive at your destination. Sometimes, people "overplan." They develop such a strict itinerary that there is no room for spontaneity. If you are confident that you will be safe and healthy while traveling to a new area, you will enjoy exploring it more. For example, if you are traveling to New Orleans on business and find yourself with a free afternoon, where would you go? If you are on a tour to Italy and your tour guide turns you loose in Florence for the day, what would you see? If you studied these destinations before you traveled, you would know that you can stroll the main streets of New Orleans's French Quarter as long as you avoid the alleys and stay where the tourists are, especially at night. You would know that a free afternoon in Florence could be enjoyed by shopping for Italian leather shoes or seeing Michelangelo's *David*, but you would also know to be wary of pickpockets. Whether traveling domestically or internationally, find out what an area has to offer to visitors and then have fun discovering these sites for yourself.

Over and over again, we have heard from travel professionals, tour guides, hotel and transportation representatives, and government agents who say that travelers are more vulnerable to crime when they are not prepared. Most of us have developed good habits at home of protecting ourselves and our belongings. We zip our purse while in crowded places, avoid dark alleys at night, and do not open our doors to strangers. However, many women will let their normal guard down when they travel. Somehow, there is a tendency to think that nothing can happen to us when we are traveling, especially when we go on vacation. Unfortunately, this is not always the case, and we do need to develop habits of protecting ourselves wherever we go. The good news is that once these habits are developed and you become aware of potential dangers, you can avoid those dangers without living in fear.

Knowing what to expect when traveling to a new area, especially to foreign countries, will also prepare you to observe and enjoy lifestyles that are vastly different from ours. It will also help you to understand and be prepared when you visit areas where freedom may be more restrictive than what we are used to in the United States. For those who have not traveled in countries that are experiencing political unrest, it may be alarming to see guards or police carrying automatic weapons in public places including airports. For example, on Catherine's first trip to Korea, she noted the armed soldiers at guard stations surrounding Seoul. These areas are protected 24 hours a day, and Koreans have adjusted to the sight.

Lavon had a similar experience during a trip to South America: "We disembarked the plane at the airport in Lima, Peru. Instead of going through a jetway, we had to walk on the tarmac from the plane to the airport in almost total darkness. This was a new experience for me. As we approached the terminal, I noticed that there were armed guards standing on the roof of the building as well as at the entrances. This made me apprehensive for the rest of our layover. I later found out that it was a time of heightened security and that all public venues were on alert."

When traveling to foreign destinations, a visit to the U.S. State Department website can tell you if that particular country is experiencing political unrest or if there is a travel advisory issued. You can access travel warnings directly by going to *http://travel.state.gov/travel_warnings.html* on the Internet. When traveling to destinations, in which armed guards are present in public places, do not be alarmed. Know that they are there to protect you.

Remember that it is just as important to research your domestic destination. For example, most large cities around the U.S. have areas that are definitely not safe for women to walk around or drive through, especially at night. On a road trip through the Southern states, we exited off a freeway late one evening and got lost looking for a hotel. We found ourselves in an area we felt was unsafe and as we stopped at an intersection, our car was surrounded by a group of young men roaming the streets. We were terrified because we did not know what they were doing and if we were in danger. We got out of the neighborhood as quickly as possible and vowed to read our map more closely before getting off the main streets for the rest of the trip.

Cultural Differences

It can be imperative when traveling to a foreign country to know what cultural differences will dictate how you should dress and act. Protocol is crucial in many countries around the world and women's rights are viewed differently in many cultures. If you will be traveling to a foreign country, spend some time researching the customs and protocol of that particular society. There are hand gestures that we use in the United States that may mean something harmless to us, but could be offensive when used in other cultures. It is common practice in many churches in the U.S. for women to dress casually while attending a service; however, in many churches and cathedrals around the world, you will not be allowed to enter unless you have your head and shoulders covered. While visiting a cathedral in Florence, we found there were guards at the door to make sure women had their shoulders covered. You will also be required to remove your shoes in mosques in Mid-Eastern countries and in many temples in Asian countries.

In some countries you may be asked to remove your shoes before entering a restaurant. Going unprepared can place you in an awkward situation. While in Korea, Catherine was traveling with a government delegation during the late summer when the weather was very warm. "We were attending a dinner in our honor and decided to wear long dresses; however, because it was so hot, we did not wear socks or nylons with our sandals. When we entered the restaurant, we realized we needed to remove our shoes. We did not know if it was appropriate to go barefoot without stockings and decided that we would attempt to walk to our table without anyone noticing our feet. I think we ended up making a spectacle of ourselves trying to walk and tuck our feet in at the same time!"

Many cultures have strict protocol for women doing business. When entering a room, should you shake the hand of your host? The answer is as varied as the country and culture you will be visiting. As you are researching your destination, take note of customs and protocol. There are also books and websites dedicated to helping women understand what to expect while visiting foreign countries. For example, while in Hong Kong, blinking may be considered impolite, and in Israel, a woman should not offer to shake hands but, rather, wait for her host or male companion to initiate contact.

One of our favorite websites for finding information about cultural differences is Executive Planet. You can access this website at *www.executiveplanet.com*. They provide information on "international business culture, customs and protocol, gift-giving, negotiating tactics, business entertainment, cross-cultural communication and more." You can search by country and receive tips on subjects such as how to dress for business and welcome topics of conversation. Cultural differences may go beyond just protocol issues. In Arab countries, for example, women business travelers will be accepted without veils, but only if they dress conservatively. There may actually be laws with serious consequences such as those banning women from driving in Saudi Arabia.

Personal space is viewed differently in many cultures. Americans tend to be protective of their personal space, which is usually considered an arm's length away. We usually become uncomfortable if someone stands too close while talking with us. However, in many countries it is common practice for individuals to stand very close to one another and lean in while having a conversation.

You will also want to be prepared for cultural differences that may surprise and even shock you.

Ruby Edwards, for example, who has traveled to 27 countries, tells us of a trip to Egypt in which she was traveling in a tour group. "We were touring a public building when a man approached one of the men in our group and asked if he could *buy* one of the teenage girls traveling with us! She was apprehensive for the rest of the trip."

There are also medical practices that are vastly different than we are used to in the U.S. Lavon was on a mission outreach to Argentina when she became ill. "I was so sick, that it hurt just to stand up. I spent one whole day lying in bed holding my stomach. The next morning, an older woman was summoned to the home where I was staying. She brought a jar that contained a mixture of herbs (and who knows what else) in water. She soaked a cloth in the mixture and rubbed it on my stomach. I cannot say whether it was the herbs that did the trick, but the next day I felt better!"

How to Research a Travel Destination

Understanding the culture and customs of your destination, as well as current events of the region, will help you travel with confidence. Spending a little time now will help ensure a more meaningful trip later. In this section, we will share resources and tools to help guide you. There are many resources available for finding information about travel destinations. Libraries, bookstores, travel agencies, television travel programs, and the Internet can provide history, customs, culture, and travel how-tos. Researching a travel destination does not need to be a cumbersome job. Use the resources most comfortable for you within the time you have available.

When we planned our first business trip to Washington, D.C., we looked for accommodations that were located in areas that were considered safe for out-of-town visitors. Our itinerary included a week of meetings in the core area of government offices; therefore, we looked for lodging and transportation that were convenient to our schedule. We found that staying near the Smithsonian Institution seemed to be safe because it is an area that caters to travelers. We booked a room near the museums and walked or took taxis to our meetings. We learned that, as in most cities, it is unwise to walk the streets at night and adjusted our schedule to arrive back at our hotel each day at a reasonable hour.

Once you learn how to plan travel with safety in mind, it will become easier each time you do it. Experience and knowledge will aid in making wise decisions. Find out as much about your destination as possible and ask yourself this question: "How can I keep myself safe and healthy?" As this becomes a way of thinking, it will help provide confidence to explore new destinations around the world.

Catherine has learned how to keep safety in mind while travel planning, especially when taking international trips. "I love exploring new areas and discovering the unexpected. I have walked around cities such as London, Madrid, and Sydney on my own and felt very safe because I knew some basic information about the cities before I went, such as what areas to avoid while exploring. I read books, looked on the Internet, or asked questions of locals when I arrived. If you know what to be wary of, you can travel with more confidence. You will also know ahead of time what sites you will want to see while you are there. For accommodations, I find out what types of lodging are available in the area. This allows me to have more confidence while taking a bit of a risk. I would hate to miss a wonderful travel experience because of fear of the unknown.

Several years ago, my husband Don and I were planning a combination business/pleasure trip to France, Italy, and Switzerland. We were starting out in Paris and wanted to spend a week exploring the South of France. Two months before our trip, I began to research using the Internet. To search, I would use keywords such as "France," "Mediterranean," and "Provence." One link would lead to another, so if I did not find what I was looking for on one site, I could easily find a related topic leading to a different page. One day, I came across a French travel bulletin board. A bulletin board is an Internet posting site where you can exchange messages with other Internet users. I posted a question inquiring whether anyone knew of a good hotel in Provence. I received an email from a man named

Philippe, who gave me several great suggestions. We began exchanging email, and Philippe told us that his parents rented out an apartment in their home for short stays. He sent us pictures and more details and we ended up reserving the room for seven nights. Because we did not know him, we did not give out any personal information other than our name and email address. We also had names of other hotels in the area, which we confirmed had vacancies just in case we did not feel comfortable with the situation when we arrived. We agreed to meet Philippe in Cannes and follow him to his parents' house, which was in a nearby village. We rented a car at the train station so that we would have our own transportation. When we arrived, his parents greeted us as if we were long lost friends. They were gracious and wonderful and, although they did not speak English, Philippe translated for us. The apartment was on the ground floor with a private terrace overlooking an olive grove with the Mediterranean Sea in the distance. Every evening, Philippe came over and helped with our sightseeing plans for the next day. He highlighted the areas on a map that were not-to-miss sights. We spent a most incredible week exploring the South of France.

Because this was such a positive experience, it gave me the courage to pursue private home-stays when my friend Debbie and I traveled to Great Britain recently. Through research at our local Barnes and Noble bookstore, we came across a reference to The Bulldog Club (*www.bulldogclub.com*) in London. This is a booking agency, which represents private homes open to visitors for lodging. Through them, we booked accommodations in England and Scotland. We stayed in an historic home in Hyde Park; an upscale converted tea warehouse on the Thames River, and a sixteenth century castle in Scotland. As two women traveling alone, we were unsure at first about home-stays. By taking a risk, we met delightful hosts who not only welcomed us to their homes, but also helped us plan our sightseeing tours, showed us the best places in London for tea, and directed us to incredible flea markets."

A few words of caution: Know what else is available in the region so that you have options. Do not give personal information out to people you do not know to be credible, and do not be afraid to ask for references.

Organizing Your Information

As we mentioned before, use the research methods most comfortable and convenient for you. Take notes and make lists of things you would like to see and do while traveling, as well as any advisories. One great way to approach this is to organize your information into categories.

For example, if you are traveling to London, you could begin with general information about what there is to see and do in London and then look for information about how to travel there. This information is similar to what a travel agent can provide in a destination package. Collect travel brochures, website print-outs, destination books, and other useful information. If you are adventurous and want to "explore" an area, find out how to do this safely. For example, if you want to travel to Tuscany, get a list of reputable inns or bed and breakfasts before you go. Ask your travel agent to make recommendations or go online and search for Tuscany accommodations. We searched Yahoo and found dozens of sites offering lodging. One site offered lodging at villas, farmhouses, inns, private residences, or hotels. The benefit of searching for information online, is that you can email the providers of these services and ask specific questions such as whether the accommodations are in a safe area, and if they take drop-in guests.

Useful Resources

Internet

The Internet is one of the most comprehensive tools you can use to research a destination, especially when you are considering safety issues. Through the Internet, you can see pictures and obtain critical information that will aid in your travel planning. If you are Internet savvy, you can "surf" through websites designed to aid in travel planning. Begin by using keywords such as "travel." This will give you access to hundreds of sites specific to the travel industry. Use destination-specific keywords when searching, such as "London" or "Atlanta." These will usually provide listings from travel bureaus or visitor associations that can tell you about the area including history, maps, accommodations, and transportation.

Websites, such as Expedia at *www.expedia.com*, can help you in choosing travel services. There is a search engine that can lead you to departments designed to help you with specific travel needs. We love Expedia's Family Travel Community at *http://communities.msn.com/ExpediaFamilyTravel.* This site will give you information ranging from tips for taking the kids on the plane to how to chat with other families online.

Other sites such as *www.journeywoman.com* are designed specifically for women travelers. Journeywoman™ provides travel information and tips, as well as shares experiences of their readers. There are usually additional links from these sites that can lead you to other web pages.

Another website focused on women is Her Mail, located at *www.hermail.net.* This site is an international directory of women travelers. It is a free email-based service designed to connect women who are traveling to different parts of the world and are interested in knowing about that area before arriving. You can find contacts of women in many destinations who can give you first-hand advice about their area.

Women business travelers should check out the website *www.womenbusinesstravelers.com*, which focuses on the woman business traveler and the concerns she may encounter while traveling, such as where to dine if she needs to entertain a client. For example, you can go to their concierge page and find such tips as how to choose restaurants and find the best entertainment, all with the perspective of women business travelers.

When researching online, start out with a search engine such as *www.google.com* and type in keywords such as "travel women." You will receive a list of sites designed for women interested in a variety of travel information.

Airline websites such as United Airlines at *www.united.com/* have pages showing maps of major airports and travel support. Airlines are also now offering travel tips; for example, Delta's website at *www.delta.com/* offers advice for choosing airline seats for infants and toddlers.

Want to know if you can use your hair dryer at the hotel in Barbados? Check out Steve Kropla's website at *http://www.kropla.com/* for information about electricity around the world and what adapters will be needed to access plug-ins.

TravelingSafe.com is our website designed to provide travel safety information. You can access the site at any time at *www.travelingsafe.com* and find a weekly safety tip and links to other travel-related websites.

We recommend Ronald and Caryl Krannich's book, *Travel Planning on the Internet: The Click and Easy Guide*™ (Impact Publications, 2001). This comprehensive guidebook lists over 2,000 travel-related websites along with descriptions of what is found on each site and virtually covers every aspect of travel planning. It includes basic Internet search techniques and how to find everything from airline safety records to worldwide holidays that may affect your travel plans. Their own website, *www.ishoparoundtheworld.com,* provides destination information and travel tips based on their series of guidebooks, *Treasures and Pleasures of...Best of the Best.*

When researching destinations on the Internet, look at maps of the area and download pictures. Follow links that will tell you about the history, what there is to see and do while you are there, and what accommodations are available. Many hotels will not only list amenities, but will also show actual pictures of their accommodations. Be aware, however, that it is common for hotels to spend more money decorating the lobby and that a beautiful reception area does not necessarily reflect a beautiful guestroom. If available, follow the links that will show an actual picture of the room you are choosing.

Also note that pictures may not always depict an accurate reflection of the surrounding area. Leonard and Anne Grubowski, for example, found a hotel in Greece that promised a splendid view of the Acropolis, however, when they arrived, their hotel room overlooked a giant advertisement billboard hiding the view of the Acropolis somewhere behind.

If you are not sure about an area or what is listed on the Internet, email or call with specific questions. Keep your itinerary in mind as you search: What types of services will you be using? Will you need accommodations, transportation, or business services? Combine your specific needs with the habit of asking questions about safety and health for travelers. You will travel with more confidence if you gain as much information as possible about an area before you go.

Libraries

Your library can be an invaluable travel resource. Trained staff can assist you in locating specific information. Besides books, libraries stock videos, audiotapes, magazines, newspapers, and government directories. If you do not have access to the Internet at home or work, visit your local library, as most now offer online services to the public. Check to make sure the travel books and videos are up to date, as it can be critical to have current information, especially when traveling internationally. If you have Internet access at home, you can most likely log on to your local library. Follow the directions to search for books on the subject of travel and women. Most libraries that are now online offer email response to specific questions.

We emailed our local library and asked for information for women travelers. They responded within 48 hours with recommendations on what types of publications would fit our request. They told us they had books and articles on women traveling, women traveling alone, and women traveling for business. They have books classified by travel location and books with information such as safe places for women to stay and eat while in Rome. They also referred us to their online magazine with articles and their electronic resources site which provides links to other websites focused on women travelers.

Library staff can direct you to books focusing on other women's issues that may be travel related. You may want to pick up a book on self-defense for women to understand things you can do to protect yourself. Remember to look in the health section to find books on the kinds of food preferable while on the road, and on eating lightly while traveling.

Bookstores

Many bookstores today offer a relaxed environment in which you can browse through books at leisure. It is popular now for many bookstores to include a coffee bistro that offers drinks and pastries to enjoy while reviewing your choices. You will find a wide range of publications that are destination-specific and can assist you in planning where to go, what to see, and where to stay.

Most large bookstores have a travel section organized by country or travel topic. If you are traveling to Paris, for example, you will find guides on sightseeing, accommodations, and transportation. The popular guides such as *Fodors Travel Publications, Arthur Frommer's Budget Travel*, and *Eyewitness Travel Guides* are some of the best resources for destination information. You will find books that address the history, culture, and customs of many foreign countries. Small paperback books offer the convenience of taking the book with you when you travel for quick reference. Most larger bookstores have a special section on women's issues including health and safety. Look here for guides to healthy eating around the world. You may also find audiotapes such as those for learning a foreign language. If you are planning a trip to Mexico, you might want to brush up on your Spanish. Many residents of foreign countries appreciate visitors who try to speak their language.

Newspapers—Travel Section

There is a travel section in most local Sunday papers that is a wealth of information. It lists the latest and sometimes best airfares, as well as, the current temperature and forecast for many major cities around the world. Most travel sections contain a feature destination, usually one that is in the U.S. and then one that is international. You might look to this venue to find travel clubs and forums for women that are held in your area. This is a great source for keeping up with the latest travel news year around.

Travel Publications

If you subscribe to a magazine that is focused on destination travel, you will be able to research destinations with every new edition. *Condé Nast Traveler* magazine is a great example of a publication which provides destination information around the world. Usually travel writers will give you a personal look into local culture when describing a destination and will, most likely, even tell you the negative aspects of an area. Travel publications are rich with the latest information about destinations and tips for many types of travel consumers such as adventure travel or senior travel.

There are also many women's magazines that, while not specifically travel publications, include articles about places around the world, as well as special trips designed for women that may include shopping at private antique sales and afternoon tea at a world-class hotel. These types of tours for women can be much safer than traveling on your own and less stressful because the planning is done for you.

Embassies, Consulates, and State Department

When traveling to foreign countries, it is important to know of any travel advisory warnings which may be in effect in that particular country and immunizations and travel documents required for entry.

Don't assume that the beautiful travel brochures will describe any dangers that might confront an unsuspecting tourist. For example, as Catherine was planning a trip to Indonesia, she accessed the U.S. State Department website to find out more about the country. She discovered that the State Department had issued a warning advising U.S. citizens to avoid travel to Indonesia at the time. There had been a rash of terrorist bombings in the area due to extreme political unrest. The stack of brochures on her desk were silent on the subject.

You can access up-to-date information from embassies and consulates of foreign governments, or the U.S. State Department. These are accessible at your library or through the Internet. Most libraries carry a publication called *Congressional Directory*, which will list the address of your selected embassy.

We recommend accessing the U.S. State Department through their website, *www.state.gov/,* for information about foreign countries. One of the sites through the U.S. State Department is *www.state.gov/www/background_notes,* which provides some of the most current and factual resources. This is the web address for the *Background Notes* page where you can search your destination country and receive an official profile of that country. The profile includes: People, Government, Economy, Religion, History, Political Conditions, Travel, and Business Information.

Another recommended site for crime and security information, areas of instability, and required travel documents, is *http:/ /travel.state.gov/travel_warnings.html*. This will provide you with a Consular Information Sheet.

Travel Agencies

Researching your travel destination can be time consuming and may not be convenient for your schedule. There are professionals who have already done the work for you. Travel agencies are one of the most comprehensive sources for providing travel information. Ask your travel agent for brochures, maps, and sightseeing pamphlets about your destination. Many agencies will provide a destination package for you. They can also be a source of travel advisories for problem areas. Ask to speak to agents who have traveled to the area. They can give you more specific information. Ask especially if they have women agents who have traveled to the place you want to go. Ask them specific questions such as whether they felt safe as a woman traveling there or did they have any problems. We have gathered a wealth of information from women who are well traveled and have told us what to be aware of while traveling to certain destinations. Whether traveling independently or on tours, your travel agent can arrange your itinerary, make reservations for you, and provide information about your trip. Be sure to use reputable agencies with experienced agents who are either well traveled themselves or are experts at finding comprehensive information for you. Ask people you know who have traveled for recommendations of agencies, or check with your local Better Business Bureau to find out if there have been any complaints against the company.

Personal Recommendations

Friends, family, and co-workers can provide first-hand experience of travel destinations. Ask for specific recommendations and be sure to ask what was great, as well as what were the negative aspects of their trip. Ask them what airline and ground transportation they used; where they stayed; and what areas they visited. Also ask them if they had any problems with safety and, if so, how they dealt with it. Take notes as you talk with them. Incorporate their experiences and knowledge into your travel planning. Keep in mind, though, that just because Aunt Martha was mugged in New York City does not mean that it is a dangerous destination or that because a co-worker got sick in Mexico, you cannot eat the food there. Rather, learn from others experiences how to keep yourself safe and healthy.

If you will be traveling out of the country, you can contact a local church of the nationality you are researching to glean information about the culture. Many times, local churches will have English-speaking staff who have moved to the U.S. from foreign countries. Use personal experiences with your other research in order to get a truer picture of the destination you are interested in.

Researching Cruises

Cruises are a unique entity, as they are in a sense a destination while at the same time providing transportation *and* accommodations. Cruises can be a safe way for women to travel because they provide a group atmosphere in a contained area for most of the trip. You can tour ports in groups for safety and find a variety of activities onboard with other passengers. The all-inclusive rates will allow you to limit the amount of money you need to take with you. However, there have been horror stories from women who have taken cruises. Incidents ranging from rapes and thefts while onboard, to purse snatching while visiting ports, have caused concern for safety. We suggest that you find a good cruise travel agent who can recommend a reputable cruise line. A good resource is Cruise Lines International Association (CLIA). Cruise companies must adhere to strict rules to be a CLIA member.

> Cruise Lines International Association
> 500 Fifth Avenue, Suite 1407
> New York, NY 10110
> Phone: 212- 921-0066
> Website: *www.cruising.org*

When researching cruises, look for safety and health records for particular cruise lines. You can find "Sanitation and Inspections of International Cruise Ships" reports from the Centers for Disease Control and Prevention's international traveler's hotline at 1-877-FYI-TRIP (1-877-394-8747), via their autofax service at 1-888-CDC-FAXX (1-888-232-3229), or their Internet home page at *www.cdc.gov/travel/* (follow the link to *Cruise Ships*)

For a *Cruise Ship Consumer Fact Sheet*, access the U.S. Coast Guard website at *www.uscg.mil/hq/g-m/cruiseship.htm.* This will provide information on how cruise ships are regulated by the U.S. Coast Guard and other U.S. government agencies, including the International Convention for the Safety of Life at Sea (referred to as SOLAS).

We found some great cruising tips at *www.concierge.com* that would be worth checking out before you go. This site, featuring *Conde Nast Traveler*, provides resources on choosing cruises and has sections with information on tipping and cruise disputes. Follow the link to *Cruise Guide*.

Cruise Opinion, *www.cruiseopinion.com*, is a great site for researching cruise information because you can access a huge database of reviews submitted by people who have taken cruises. You can search reviews by specific cruise line and receive detailed opinions of their experiences such as cleanliness, safety, food service, and more.

Cruise Critic, *www.cruisecritic.com*, is a site that contains a community of member reviews of different cruise lines. You can also search for reviews of the specific line you are interested in. The *New Member Reviews* contain up-to-date opinions posted for a variety of cruise experiences on different vessels.

Again, we recommend that you talk with an expert cruise travel agent who can "fit" a cruise to your specific travel criteria. For example, we read several cruise reviews from passengers who wanted a quiet, safe, cruise experience and found that they had booked a cruise that included a corporate group who practically took over the whole ship, and were loud and annoying to other passengers. Other passengers shared tales of illnesses from eating food during port visits. Tell your travel agent that you are a female traveler concerned for safety and health and request information about the particular cruise line, such as whether sprinklers are in the cabins and public areas.

Find more information about staying safe on cruises in Chapter Eight, "Your Personal Safety Guide."

Your Specific Travel Needs

As you begin to plan your travel, take into consideration *how* you travel. For example, do you have needs that may hinder access to some places? Are you traveling with children? Are you a senior traveling alone? These considerations will be important as you gather information about your destination.

Traveling for Business

Thousands of women travel each year for business both domestically and internationally, and predictions are that women will continue to constitute a large section of the business travel market. When traveling for business, your destination will probably not be up to you; however, it is still important for you to find out all the information you can about where you will be traveling. If your company has offices in the area you will be traveling to, call female employees and ask for recommendations. Their experiences can be some of the most valuable information you will gain before traveling.

Look on the Internet for maps of the area and visit websites of local visitors associations. These websites can help orient you with an area so that you will feel more comfortable when you arrive. Call or write to the city or visitors association and ask questions about where the safest areas are for women travelers and safe methods of local transportation. Network with women's groups where you can gain valuable information from other seasoned business travelers.

Traveling With Children

Taking children on a trip brings a whole new challenge for the traveling woman. Whether attending a convention in which you are bringing along the family, or taking an annual vacation, traveling with children can be fun but can also be strenuous. Not only does a mother have to keep track of her own belongings, but she also has to care for her child and his/her health and safety as well. An airport public relations agent told us that one of the easiest targets for criminals looking for a purse to snatch is a mother with a young child. The mother is usually trying to carry the child or hold his hand, manage a diaper bag, carry-on, and purse on her shoulder and sometimes even trying to drag an infant seat along. Trying to manage to get through an airport with a child is not an easy task and can lead to carelessness with items such as purses, which can end up tossed over her back, tempting to a thief.

Long drives in the car, interruption in eating schedules, and standing in long lines at airports are just some of the considerations to plan for when traveling with children. There are a variety of travel books and guides written specifically for traveling with children. If you are researching on the Internet, use a search engine such as *www.yahoo.com* and use keywords such as "travel" and "children." You will find a variety of sites providing information on everything from how to keep kids happy on airplanes to what documents the U.S. State Department requires before taking children out of the country.

Talking with your child's doctor can arm you with tips such as how to deal with the interruption in sleep patterns while traveling. Bookstores such as Barnes and Noble and Borders have travel sections where you can find a variety of books on travel-ing with children. Call or log on to travel product suppliers such as Magellan's Travelers' Catalog at *www.magellans.com* for products such as Earplanes, an earplug to help reduce ear pain for children while taking off and landing.

Senior Women Travelers

If you are a senior woman, there are many options for choos-ing travel destinations. Hundreds of tour companies are avail-able throughout the U.S. that cater to the senior traveler. Begin by deciding what type of travel you would like to do, such as traveling to warm climates with relaxed activities or touring museums in Europe. Group travel may be one of the safer choices for senior women. Your activities will be pre-planned and you can have a choice of sharing accommodations.

A great place to start in your destination research is the American Association of Retired Persons (AARP):

> 601 E Street, NW
> Washington, DC 20049
> Phone: 1-800-424-3410 or 202-434-2277
> Website: www.aarp.org

They have a variety of travel discounts for members and can provide information on issues such as Medicare coverage. (It is critical to know what your insurance covers while travel-ing – see more in Chapter Five, "Staying Healthy While Trav-eling.")

If you are connected to the Internet, there are hundreds of sites that focus on senior women. One such site is Senior Women

Web located at *www.seniorwomen.com*. We especially like their travel section and the letters from other readers describing destinations they have visited.

Female Student Travelers

Student travelers represent a large segment of the female travel industry. Most student travelers will be traveling as part of an organized school program with staff to assist with travel questions. However, many female student travelers we interviewed were not savvy about safety issues. We interviewed half a dozen young women in Paris who had their purses or wallets stolen within hours of arriving in the country. They told us they were not prepared with the knowledge of how to protect their belongings. Precautions, such as keeping their purses in front of them and carrying their money and passports in a money belt, could have prevented the thieves from getting to their valuables. The concern of student travel from a safety standpoint is that students will usually need to travel on a small budget that requires staying in hostels and using public transportation.

If traveling on a study-abroad program, take care in researching the area in which you will be staying, keeping safety in mind as you plan. Check out websites such as the Rough Guides at *www.roughguides.com* for travel networking and advice.

The ISIC Association produces and regulates an International Student Identity Card (ISIC) that can help provide identity and discounts for student travelers. The association distributes the card within local territories that are listed on the website *www.istc.org/p_ab_isic.asp*. The card is recognized in over 90 countries, and many institutions will honor discounts. They also have a 24-hour emergency multilingual assistance service. In the U.S. you can purchase the ISIC cards through *www.counciltravel.com.*

The International Student Travel Confederation is a confederation of student organizations around the world whose focus is to develop, promote, and facilitate travel among young people and students. You can access their website at *www.istc.org.* Call or write to them at:

> International Student Travel Confederation
> Herengracht 479
> 1017 BS Amsterdam
> The Netherlands
> Tel: +31 20 421 28 00 , Fax: +31 20 421 28 10

With females representing approximately 40 percent of the more than 60 million U.S. citizens traveling abroad annually, it is imperative for us to learn how to keep ourselves safe and healthy while away from home. Understanding our destination and being armed with the knowledge of how to protect ourselves will help ensure a safer and more rewarding travel experience.

2

Choosing Safe Transportation

From airlines to taxis, transportation planning is one of the most important aspects of travel safety. While there are no guarantees against unforeseen accidents, becoming educated will help assure a safer trip. Using reputable transportation providers is imperative! For example, if you require public transportation when you arrive at your destination, make sure you know how to recognize reputable companies before you go. As you gather your luggage or clear customs, it is easy to get disoriented about how to find local transportation to your hotel. It is common, especially in foreign countries for men to swarm passengers as soon as they get out of the luggage area and offer taxi service. Most airports will have kiosks or desks for ground transportation information where you can obtain information on how to get authorized taxi or bus service.

Many travelers, especially international travelers, will use a variety of transportation. You may fly to your destination, use a taxi to get to your hotel, ride the subway to a meeting, and take a tour bus to see the sights. Each time you board an airplane, get into a taxi, or climb onto a tour bus, you are putting your trust in the person operating the controls. It is important that you choose transportation providers carefully.

According to Rochelle Sobel, founder of the Association for Safe International Road Travel (ASIRT), "Statistics indicate that the number one cause of accidental deaths of Americans traveling abroad is road traffic accidents." Rochelle's son, Aron, was killed in a bus accident in Turkey in 1995. A University of Maryland medical student, Aron was doing his final rotation abroad. He planned to spend four days in Turkey before coming home to graduate. He boarded a bus that was returning from the coast and, according to survivors, the driver was speeding down the wrong lane and had just exited a dark tunnel on a road that had been designated as unsafe. The "death curve" had no guardrails and was in a mountainous area where tourists frequented. "People had asked the bus driver to slow down," said Sobel, "and he didn't. He hit oncoming traffic and the whole bus careened down a ravine." Aron was killed along with 22 other people, including the bus driver.

As a result of her son's death, Rochelle became aware of the need for education about international road safety. Through ASIRT, she has worked tirelessly to promote awareness of road safety issues in countries around the world. Organizations such as ASIRT are valuable resources to use while planning your trip. (You can access their website at *www.asirt.org*)

As you search for transportation, consider all the types of transportation you will need on your trip. For example, if you are traveling by air, determine the best way to get to your hotel from the airport. There are cities in which it can be very safe to take public transportation such as subways to and from the airport, while at other destinations this can be risky because of pickpockets who target visitors. If you are going to be met by someone, arrange a meeting place ahead of time to avoid confusion. If you do not know the person, ask for identifying characteristics. Don't rely only on a sign that they may hold with your name on it, or be placed in the position of wandering around the airport looking for them. Unfortunately, thieves hang out at airports as well as other public places and know how to recognize a viable target. They will opt for the easiest target to rob: usually a traveler who is distracted or overburdened with bags and not paying attention to all of his/her belongings. They know how to slip a hand into an open purse or carry-on bag that is carelessly tossed over the shoulder. The best defense is to be prepared before you go by knowing what type of transportation you will need and how to find it.

Choosing Transportation Wisely

Airline Travel Safety

In the last few years, headlines reporting air accidents have increased the concern for airline safety. We want to be assured that when we board an aircraft, we will arrive safely at our destination. Even though you are not in control of the safety of the aircraft, there are precautions you can take when choosing a carrier.

Consider airline safety records: There are resources available, such as AirSafe.com that will help you make an educated decision before you book your flight. This is especially important when flying internationally and traveling on foreign airlines.

According to some reports, the Federal Aviation Administration (FAA), which regulates U.S. airlines, performs some direct inspections of overseas carriers that fly to the U.S., but primarily relies on foreign authorities to regulate their airlines. The agency also assesses whether foreign governments meet international aviation safety standards, but it has limited power to police foreign airlines. Therefore, it can be imperative that you understand the safety record of airlines before you fly. AirSafe.com provides information ranging from airline safety records to how to be safe during turbulence. You can access their website at *www.AirSafe.com* or call them at 206-300-8727.

Choice of airline carriers: When traveling internationally, your choice of airline carriers will be limited to your particular destination. For example, you may have ten choices of carriers from the U.S. to England while you may have fewer choices traveling to Taiwan. Researching safety records of the available airlines will assist you in making an informed decision.

Other factors which need to be considered:

Departure and arrival times: Your schedule should coincide with the safest times to be at your destination. If possible, avoid arriving late at night. Review your flight itinerary carefully, paying close attention to your arrival, departure, and layover schedule.

Your itinerary may not be in your control: Another party, such as your employer or foreign host, may be making travel arrangements on your behalf. They may book your reservations according to available airline flights or work schedules. If possible, request a travel itinerary suitable for your safety needs.

Confirming flight itinerary: Most airlines require you to call 24 to 72 hours prior to departure to confirm your flight itinerary. Check with your reservation agent when booking flights. You *must* confirm your return flights when traveling internationally. Also, ask the agent what terminal your flight will be departing from. In some major airports, there may be up to six or seven terminals that are usually far apart. Some are far enough apart that you will need to take a shuttle or walk for up to 30–40 minutes to get to the next terminal. This delay could cause you to miss your flight, so make sure you check which terminal you will be departing from before you go to the airport.

Paper Ticket vs. Electronic Ticketing: When you purchase an airline ticket, you may have a choice between the traditional paper ticket or an electronic ticket. There are pros and cons for each method and you will need to consider your specific travel itinerary and choose accordingly.

Some pros and cons:

Paper tickets are easier to use in instances when you need to change flight schedules at the last minute or get bumped. If the airline computer system is down or encountering problems, a paper ticket makes checking in easier. Some airlines require paper tickets to check luggage all the way through on some international flights. Some negative aspects are that paper tickets can be difficult to replace if lost or stolen and you must keep track of paper tickets while traveling.

Electronic tickets can make check-in easier and faster. You do not have to keep track of a paper ticket while traveling, although airlines recommend keeping a copy of your flight itinerary, so you will carry a paper document anyway. Electronic ticketing can make booking reservations over the Internet easier because you do not have to wait for a paper ticket to be mailed to you. Electronic tickets may make it easier to change flights over the phone.

We have used paper and electronic tickets for traveling both domestically and internationally. While we like the ease of electronic ticketing, we recommend paper tickets for trips when you will be changing planes often with close connections, especially internationally. Also if you are traveling domestically during peak traveling times, or traveling during seasons when weather can cause flight delays and you may have to change flights quickly, paper tickets may be more convenient because you can sometimes take them to other airlines and they will honor them. This is changing with the advance of electronic transfer, so ask your airline agent when making reservations what type of ticket would be best for your itinerary.

Driving

Driving away from home can be a challenge if you are not familiar with the roads or if you encounter unfavorable weather patterns. If you plan on driving, whether taking your own car or renting a car, take into consideration the weather and road conditions at your destination.

Lavon has enjoyed traveling throughout the southern United States and has experienced torrential rains and fog as thick as "pea soup!" "In some places, it can rain more in three hours than many states experience in a month! I have learned to make sure that my windshield wipers work well, and that the tires on the vehicle are in good shape."

One of the most important safety items to have while traveling by car is a good map. Women can be especially vulnerable if they get lost in areas prone to crime. Search your route before you go if possible. Access websites such as Yahoo at *www.yahoo.com*, click on maps, and you can get driving directions for domestic destinations. You can also access www.*mapquest.com* to obtain driving directions within the U.S. and Canada as well as Europe. When traveling domestically we suggest you obtain a good road atlas. You can find them in most bookstores or places such as AAA (American Automobile Association). When traveling internationally, you can find maps included in most destination-specific travel books such as *Fodors Travel Publications, Arthur Frommer's Budget Travel*, and *Eyewitness Travel Guides*. This should be one of your criteria for choosing a book on travel.

Traveling by Personal Car: If traveling in your own car, make sure that you have properly serviced your car before departure. Check the brakes, lights, tires, and windshield wipers, etc., to assure they are in good working condition. Pack an emergency car kit with you which includes a flashlight, flares, or flashing emergency light, in addition to your jack and emergency tire-changing equipment. If you will be traveling to areas in which you could experience cold weather, pack gloves, hat, and a blanket in case of emergency. We strongly recommend carrying a cell phone with you when traveling by car. It is also a good idea to have automobile travelers insurance or membership in an organization such as the American Automobile Association (AAA). Make sure you know what your insurance will and will not cover. (See more driving tips in Chapter Eight, "Your Personal Safety Guide.")

Rental Cars: The risk in renting a car while traveling is not usually with the car itself, as most rental agencies take great care in making sure that cars are well serviced and safe for drivers. The risk is that drivers are not usually aware of the laws of driving in another state and especially in foreign countries where not only laws differ greatly, but driving habits as well. A vision of leisurely driving through the wine country in France is a glorious thought to many, but attempting to navigate around the Arc de Triumph in Paris is in reality a nightmare if you are not used to driving there.

If you plan on renting a car, find out how driving laws differ in the area you will be traveling to. For example, driving under the influence of alcohol can have severe criminal penalties in many foreign countries. Driving customs also vary greatly in foreign countries; for example, you may need to know what a horn honk or a hand signal means. In some countries it is customary or even required for drivers to honk before they pass. You will also want to familiarize yourself with laws and practices regarding pedestrians, as in some countries pedestrians and bicyclists do not practice stopping at red lights as we do in the U.S.

When reserving a rental car, make sure that you know what is covered by insurance in case of an accident. Do not assume that your credit card carrier will cover the costs of repairs if you decline the rental car company's insurance coverage. Make sure your credit card covers the type of vehicle you are going to get and that it covers you in the country in which you are traveling. If you have any doubts, take the insurance that is offered by the rental agency.

Think about the size of car you need and how much you're willing to spend. Be aware that vehicle classification systems vary. The terms "compact," "mid-size," and "luxury" sometimes have different meanings among companies.

Receiving an International Driving Permit

An International Driving Permit (IDP) is a translation of your current State Driver's License. It *does not* take the place of your driver's license. IDPs are valid in over 150 countries and contain your name, photo, and driver information translated into ten languages. IDPs are not valid in an individual's country of residence. Although IDPs are not required in all countries, it is advisable to get one should you have problems while driving abroad. It will make your identification process much easier for foreign authorities.

The U.S. State Department has designated the American Automobile Association (AAA) and the American Automobile Touring Alliance (AATA) as the only authorized distributors of IDPs. To apply for an IDP, you must be at least age 18, and you will need to present two passport-size photographs and your valid U.S. license. The cost of an international driving permit from these U.S. State Department authorized organizations is $10.00. To obtain an application contact AAA or AATA by phone, fax, in person, or on the Internet.

American Automobile Association (AAA)
1000 AAA Drive

Heathrow, FL 32745-5063.
Phone: Check your local directory for offices near you
X The application is available online at
*http://www.aaamidatlantic.com/livenew/travel/
idp_form1.htm*

Or go to their homepage at *www.aaa.com* and type in
your zip code for offices near you.

American Automobile Touring Alliance (AATA)
1151 E. Hillsdale Blvd., Foster City, CA 94404,
Phone: 800-622-7070; Fax: 650-294-7105
Call for online applications through authorized
affiliates

Taxis and Limousine Service

There are many resources available to research surface transportation before you go on your trip. Many airports list transportation information on their websites. These lists often include the kind of transportation available and how to know if
these services are registered with the airport authorities. Airports almost always have agreements with taxi companies to
provide a taxi stand where the drivers are registered. London-
Heathrow Airport's website lists the names of the taxi companies and how to identify them. Upon arrival, you can inquire at
airport information or security counters how to find areas that
have taxi service. There are specific items to look for in a taxi
such as emblems painted on the door and a license with picture
identification posted on the dashboard.

Let's face it, you will not know if the driver of the taxi you
are getting into will have a safe driving record; however, you

can make sure that you choose reputable companies by knowing where to go to get a taxi. Besides airports, it is common for taxi stands to be located around larger cities. Find out what name or symbol to look for on the taxicab itself. Even if there is not a taxi stand, you can ask a restaurant host or hotel staff to call one for you, as they will know what company to use.

Limousine service is common at airports, however, they are usually much more expensive than taxis. Check the price before getting in. If you are traveling in a group, limousine service may be reasonably priced if sharing the cost, and it will most likely be a more comfortable ride than taxis. Make sure they are being hailed by the agent at the airport or by the hotel doorman, etc.

Buses

Generally speaking, the larger bus-transport organizations will offer cleaner, more reliable buses with amenities such as bathrooms. Bus companies in many underdeveloped countries will often use older, more run down buses. When buying passage on a bus, you will not always know what condition the bus will be in, so it is imperative that you use reputable providers with experienced drivers. Check with organizations such as the Association for Safe International Road Travel (ASIRT) for travel advisories and problems with providers in certain countries. There are bus companies now offering a system similar to the popular Eurorail pass. You can purchase a bus pass from the company effective for a set number of days and can get on and off when it stops in the city of your choice. It is often necessary to purchase this pass in the U.S. prior to departure.

Tour Buses: Tour buses offer one of the most affordable ways to travel. Bus systems run on a schedule allowing you to plan your travel in advance. You can also go to the concierge at your hotel and book last-minute tours to local sites. Buses also offer the convenience of pick-ups and drop-offs at a variety of places such as hotels. Tour buses can also offer a safer atmosphere for women travelers than sightseeing on their own.

The downside is that you will not be able to stop when you want and if you become ill or are uncomfortable with the driving, you will not easily be able to get on and off unless it is an emergency. While on a recent tour to Germany, Italy, and Switzerland, Catherine was on a bus in which the driver decided to take a shortcut along a narrow, winding road. Almost everyone on the bus was frightened by the time they reached their destination, not to mention very sick! "From then on, those who battled motion sickness learned to show up early for boarding and choose seats near the front of the bus!"

Although you may be more restricted, the safety of traveling with an organized group may be worth the inconvenience.

City Buses: Almost all large cities have some type of bus transport system, each offering a variety of services and features. Local buses may be intimidating for women travelers, especially if traveling alone. This will most likely not be a problem domestically, but while in a foreign country, a woman may be unsure about getting on a bus with locals. Language can be a barrier to obtaining directions for which stop to get on and off and negotiating tariffs. While other transportation, such as taxis, may have drivers used to visitors, city buses most likely are not as used to dealing with tourists, especially in foreign countries. Before traveling, find out about the local bus system at your destination to determine if this is a viable source of transportation for you. We have used local city buses in many foreign countries without a problem; however, we have always been with another person or part of a group.

If you choose to ride city buses, observe the local residents to see how they use the bus system. You may never have to show your ticket to an official; however, get caught without a ticket while riding a bus and you may be fined. If you plan on staying in a city for more than a few days and will be using buses to get around, it may be a good idea to purchase a pass that will allow multiple trips.

Subways and Trains

Many major cities have excellent subway and train systems. A little research before you go on your trip can help you find out how to access these and answer safety concerns such as what time of day is safest to travel. Many destination-specific travel books will list subway and train information. We like resources such as *Eyewitness Travel Guides* that provide schedule information and also give tips for using subways and trains. You can also request brochures by mail or from your travel agent before you go. Be prepared with a plan *before* you find yourself wandering through a subway station looking for the correct route. If you are traveling with a group, make sure everyone in your party knows the itinerary, the stop where you will disembark, your final destination, and an emergency meeting place should you get separated.

On a recent trip to Korea, for example, Catherine learned a valuable lesson in keeping everyone informed of the itinerary. "We were boarding a subway in Seoul, when suddenly the doors closed before one member of our group could get on the train.

Connie stood alone on the platform as the rest of us sped off. We were frantic at the thought that she did not know which stop we were getting off to transfer to another line. After 40 minutes we found Connie and were on our way; however from then on we developed the "Next Stop Plan." If one member of our group does not make it on the subway, everyone gets off at the next stop and waits. The person missing the train simply gets on the next train and goes to the next stop to meet up with the rest of the group."

While this may work for the subway, it may not be a viable back-up plan for other types of rail travel because some trains may be scheduled hours or even days in between. The point is, make sure you have a plan of what to do if you get separated. (Read more about protecting yourself and your belongings on subways in Chapter Eight, "Your Personal Safety Guide.")

It is very popular for students to travel through foreign countries by train. Many of these students choose to travel at night and sleep on the train. We spoke with a young college student named Natalie, who was traveling at night on a train from Amsterdam to Paris when she awoke to see a man standing over her with his hand on her luggage getting ready to pull it off the rack. She and her two female traveling companions began to yell and he immediately left. From then on, they tied their luggage to the rack or laid it under them while they slept.

Veteran travelers Leonard and Anne Grubowski, who have traveled through more than 20 countries, were warned while on a night train in Russia to keep their shoes on while sleeping, as there was a risk of having them stolen. Major name brand shoes can bring a high price on the black market.

There have also been reports that in remote places in Turkey, thieves will open a rail car door and toss in a chemical that will knock out passengers long enough for them to enter and rob travelers of their valuables. While this scenario may be the extreme, theft of valuables on trains is becoming increasingly common. When choosing rail transportation, look for cars that have locks or private "berths." Carrying a small bell with you that can be attached to the door can alert you of anyone entering your compartment. Also, we recommend carrying a small string or rope to tie luggage to a secure rack, which will prohibit easy removal of your bags.

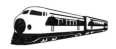

3

Booking Accommodations

Y ou close the door to your hotel room and enter a place of rest for the evening. You draw a bath and sink into the warm bubbles as thoughts of the day drift through your mind. You contemplate with excitement the experiences coming tomorrow. Maybe you reflect on notes for an important meeting, or dream of the sights and sounds you will experience as you tour a foreign city. As you rest your head on your pillow, you drift off to sleep with the comfort that you are safe and secure.

Your hotel room *should* be a safe haven while traveling. This is where you will rest and regroup, and needs to be chosen carefully. It is one of the most important decisions you will make in travel planning. In this chapter, we will explore various types of accommodations and share tips for choosing lodging with safety in mind. Knowing some basic safety precautions before you book your accommodations can help avoid potential problems.

Recently, Catherine checked into a hotel in Chicago and was given a room on the first floor where her door was facing an exit to the outside. Knowing that this was a location that could be vulnerable for a woman traveling alone, she requested a room on the second floor closer to the elevators where there would be more traffic. The hotel staff accommodated her request and apologized for the oversight saying that they normally do not place women on the first floor.

Most hotel operators today are concerned for the safety of their guests. This hotel manager had placed a traveler's safety brochure in each room to help guests become aware of good safety practices such as identifying visitors before opening their hotel room door. The American Hotel & Motel Association prints the brochure with ten traveler's safety tips that they make available for their members to place in guestrooms. Tips such as "never open your door to a stranger" and "use all locking devices" are essential practices for traveling safely.

Even with the invention of electronic locks on doors, you should always use the deadbolt lock when inside your room and never leave valuables in your room when you leave. There is now a device used by thieves called a lever-opening tool that they can slide under the door, hook onto the lever, and open the door. Many hotels have now installed a small shelf under the door lock so that this device cannot be used successfully.

Finding Accommodations

There are many factors to keep in mind as you consider your lodging needs, such as your price range, length of stay, itinerary, and transportation needs. The first issue most of us think about when considering accommodations is our price range.

This can influence the type of lodging we choose and may have an effect on our safety; however, there is no guarantee that a higher priced room means that you will be safer. There are many budget hotels that take great precautions to protect their guests. Therefore, a hotel should be chosen based on how safe and comfortable you will be during your stay.

When selecting lodging facilities, look for accommodations within your price range and then choose with safety in mind. Begin with location. Find out as much as possible about the neighborhood in which it is located. Obtain neighborhood maps and descriptions from destination-specific sources such as Internet travel sites, destination books, or brochures. If booking with an agent, ask if they have been there and what the surrounding area is like. Ask if the property is located in a well-trafficked, tourist-oriented part of town. While these areas tend to be safer, they can also be targeted areas for pickpockets and thieves. The state or country you are traveling to will also determine which areas are safer. Researching the area in which a hotel is located can be imperative in choosing safely, especially in foreign countries or in states with high crime rates.

Unfortunately, instances do sometimes occur, and we can learn from those who are willing to share their story to help us protect ourselves.

Mary Catherine, who has traveled through 30 states and many foreign countries on business, was the victim of a man who followed her to her hotel room. Mary Catherine writes about her experience while staying at a hotel in Illinois where an unknown intruder followed her into her hotel room, tied her up and tried to strangle her. "It was the last room on the floor, and the only occupied room that night on that floor. I believe it was an employee, as he had a bathrobe sash to tie me up with, a pillowcase to put over my head and rubber gloves on. He tackled me from behind. As we went down, I began pinching his testicles, which I continued to do until he managed to get my hands tied. Because I was screaming ("Fire" - to no one else on the floor), he stuffed a piece of clothing into my mouth. When I bit him I realized he had rubber gloves on. He got up, and I got untied. He tied me up again and I tried to pinch his testicles again. This happened twice more, at which time he took a T-shirt and tied it around my neck. He strangled me with the arms of the T-shirt until I almost passed out. Then I quit struggling, and he stopped strangling me. Then he left. Luckily, the only injuries I suffered were scratches and bruises, and hemorrhaging in my eyes. He was never apprehended." When asked how her traveling habits have changed, Mary Catherine says, "I am much more careful about where my room is in relation to exits, and I will not take a ground floor room or one at the end of the hall. I also watch for suspicious persons as I enter my room." She adds, "Based on probabilities, I will not have another encounter like I had. I am more careful and don't put myself into dangerous situations. In general, most hotels try to take the proper precautions. I worked as a hotel manager for 10 years, so when I see lapses in security, I point them out without hesitation. If I don't feel comfortable, I will find another place to stay."

While most of us will never experience problems like this while traveling, it is important to take steps to help ensure safety. When given a choice, ask for a room near an elevator, as this can be safer because there will be more people around. Avoid rooms near hotel exits or on lower floors that may make you vulnerable to intruders. Think of your itinerary such as: Will there be a need for you to walk from your hotel to a parking lot, taxi stand, or bus stop? Will your schedule require going out at night? Will you be alone or traveling with someone?

Booking Ahead vs. Spontaneity

Most likely, if you are traveling for business, you will have pre-scheduled appointments and it will be necessary to have accommodations arranged before you leave on your trip. If traveling for leisure, however, you may be tempted to explore an area and spontaneously stop for the night. You can do this safely by knowing some general information before you go. Make a list of reputable lodging properties while planning your trip. You can print a list of properties from the Internet or get small lodging guides. Carry this with you for reference. This will allow the freedom to explore an area and stop whenever you feel like it while at the same time, provide an assurance of finding safe accommodations for the night.

Fire Safety

When looking for accommodations, another safety concern is protection against fires. Throughout the U.S., we do not often hear of hotel fires mainly because of our strict codes. However, fire codes for lodging facilities differ greatly throughout the world. This should be taken into consideration when choosing accommodations, especially in Third World countries where poor or nonexistent fire protection exists.

If you are traveling to an area in which the quality of accommodations is unknown, don't be afraid to ask about fire safety protection. Ask questions such as whether smoke alarms and fire sprinklers are installed in guest rooms. Most reputable hotels will have emergency exit routes posted on the back of the guestroom door.

We suggest that when you put together your safety kit, you include a battery-operated smoke detector and flashlight. Be sure to place the smoke detector in a high place and away from air conditioners and air ducts. Sharper Image sells their Travel Companion®, an alarm clock, bedside flashlight, smoke detector, and motion sensor, all in one, for just under $60. You can access their website at *www.sharperimage.com* or call 1-800-344-4444. For travel flashlights, TravelSmith.com has a Palm-Size Flashlight/Lantern for $14 that you can carry in your palm, hang on a nail, or set on a table. Their toll-free number is 1-800-950-1600. Magellan's Travelers' Catalog carries a similar flashlight, and if you will be traveling to areas where you are concerned about fire protection, check out their Evac-U8 Smoke Hood. This small container opens into a hood that will protect you for up to 20 minutes from smoke and toxic gases. Cost is just under $70. Their website is *www.magellans.com,* or call 1-800-962-4943.

If there is a fire in the hotel, here are a few tips that may help to save your life:

- Feel the door to see if it is hot and, if it is, **do not open**. If the door is cold you should open it slowly and if smoke comes in close it quickly.

- If you can leave the room by the door, go quickly to the escape route you have already checked out. **Do not use the elevator**.

- If you cannot exit through the door, stay close to the floor while looking for other avenues of escape.

- If you have a window that opens and you are no higher than the second floor you may choose to jump. Don't try jumping out any higher than that, as you may be seriously injured.

- If the window is not an option, try to signal the firemen that you are in the room. Maybe putting a sheet out the window or, if the window won't open, you could use your lipstick to put a message on the window. Then go to the bathroom and wet down everything you can such as towels, sheets, etc. and put them around the room at all the cracks and areas where the smoke can get into your room.

Remember that most people who die in fires are actually killed by smoke inhalation.

Types of Lodging

Hotels

Hotels throughout the world differ greatly in their amenities and guest safety programs. Keep in mind that the three-star hotel you are accustomed to in the United States may not be the same three star hotel in a foreign country. Beds in foreign countries are also not what you may be used to. It is common to have two twin beds pushed together when requesting a room for two. Becoming familiar with the hotel rating systems available will help. Look closely at the listings of amenities and pay attention to location. Hotel quality even varies from state to state, so always find out as much as you can about the hotel when you make reservations. Don't be afraid to ask about security precautions such as whether they lock all outside doors after 9:00pm, etc.

Richard Ransome, general manager of the Sheraton Airport Hotel in Portland, Oregon, encourages choosing name brand hotels while traveling. "There is usually a set of standards that the name encourages even if hotels are franchised," he states. Richard, who has been in the hotel business for over 25 years, says that many companies require that all their hotels have a written security program and that owners and general managers are responsible for establishing and maintaining a safe and secure environment. Look for other security requirements when requesting hotel rooms such as: Do doors have both a primary and secondary locking device? Do room doors have a one-way door viewer? Are keys re-coded after each guest? Richard has also noticed an increase in women ordering room service for safety reasons. This should be considered when making your hotel reservation. If you are traveling alone and are not comfortable with eating out, choose a hotel with a restaurant.

What to look for in a guestroom:

- Located near an elevator on 2nd–4th floor
- Double locks, preferably a bar lock
- One-way viewer on the door
- Smoke detectors

Keep in mind that standards vary throughout the world and you may not have the same security devices in foreign hotels as in domestic hotels. Even name brand hotels in foreign countries do not necessarily guarantee the same quality as domestic hotels. Do not be afraid to ask what safety precautions hotels employ to protect their guests.

When choosing hotels, begin with a list of your needs by considering these questions:

- How much time will you spend at the hotel?
- Are there business or office amenities you will need?
- Do they provide shuttle service?
- Do you need close access to public transportation?
- Is there a restaurant in the hotel or close by?

Next, ask questions about safety:

- Where is the hotel located? (In business or tourist area)
- Are there double locks on the room doors?
- Is there a one-way door viewer?
- Can you reserve a specific guestroom location such as away from exits and above the first floor?
- Is the parking area close to the hotel entrance and well lit?
- If located in inner city, do they have valet parking?

Remember when asking about location to look for hotels in areas that cater to tourists and business travelers. Well-traveled streets, busy shops and restaurants may provide a safer surrounding than a remote location. You will also have better access to transportation.

Motels

The difference between a hotel and motel is that in a hotel you will normally enter your room through a lobby and inside corridor, while in a motel the room is usually accessed from outside. Newer motels are changing their design, however, and building them with inside corridors. Hotels will usually have restaurant facilities, while most motels do not offer this amenity. Motels can be a more economical way to travel; however, women travelers can be more vulnerable. When choosing motels, look for reputable businesses with good security programs. Since rooms are usually facing or near the parking lot, make sure the parking area is well lit and free from large bushes that someone could hide behind. Ask for a room near the front office, and make sure there are strong locks on room doors. Avoid rooms with connecting doors to other guestrooms if traveling alone. Don't be afraid to tell the reservations agent that you are a woman traveler and concerned about safety.

Bed and Breakfasts

A Bed and Breakfast traditionally refers to a private home that provides lodging and breakfast included in one price. B&Bs can range from small homes to larger historic buildings. The term "B&B" is now commonly used to describe any lodging facility that includes breakfast in the arrangement. Bed and Breakfasts are very popular in many foreign countries and may offer a safe alternative for women travelers. B&Bs provide not only the opportunity to experience native culture, but also an environment in a family setting which may give you peace of mind. In Great Britain, it is common to find small signs along the road advertising B&B accommodations. Catherine and her friend Debbie experienced many B&B stays while traveling throughout this area. Tempting as it might be to act adventurous and stop when you "feel like it," it is not the best choice with safety in mind, unless you carry a list of reputable properties. You can obtain lists of available Bed and Breakfasts ahead of time and make reservations or carry the list with you so that you know where to look when you want to stop for the night. Look on the

Internet or ask your travel agent for a B&B guide in the area in which you will be traveling. You can also stop at a local tourist bureau who can recommend places to stay and can sometimes make the call for you to check last-minute availability. Again, don't be afraid to ask questions about safety provisions; how-

 ever, keep in mind that these are private homes and most likely will not offer the same amenities as a major hotel. They should have locking doors and safe, well-lit parking areas. Your arrival and departure times will be stricter than at a hotel, and you may not be able to come and go as freely during your stay; however, the advice about the local area and the security of staying with a family are usually well worth the restrictions.

Richard Ransome, who is from England, says that he prefers B&Bs in the country as opposed to those located in large cities. His experience is that most B&Bs in the larger cities are located in remote areas on small streets that may not be as secure as a hotel location. While the actual property may be safe to stay, getting to and from the B&B may be risky for women. B&Bs are his choice of accommodations for safety while traveling in the countryside. "I think they are definitely the way to go and usually very safe for women travelers."

Inns

An inn is a small hotel with a restaurant that offers full meal service in addition to breakfast. The restaurant may also serve people who are non-lodging guests. Inns are very similar to Bed and Breakfasts in that they are often family owned and operated. They can provide a safe and secure place to stay for women. In addition to the quaintness and charm, the atmosphere is very often more family oriented and can provide a sense of security missing from a hotel room. Inns can be located in the country as a converted family home or in a major city as a small hotel property. As with B&Bs or any lodging facility, choose inns by looking for guidebooks or Internet resources which lists inns with recommendations or rating systems. Look for safety issues such as parking in well-lit areas and safe neighborhoods, as well as good locks on bedroom doors.

Hostels

Hostels are very popular with students and backpackers. Most hostels offer nothing more than a bed for the night although some also offer a continental breakfast. A typical hostel will have dormitory-style rooms with beds and lockers for storing your valuables. The beds will usually have a mattress but no bedding. Many hostels offer sheets and towels that you can rent for a small fee. The toilet and shower are usually down the hall. It is not uncommon for the electrical outlet for hair dryers to be located in the hallway. Hostels are an extremely economical way to travel; however, if not chosen carefully they can be a risk, especially for women travelers. When choosing hostels, get a list of reputable properties before you travel. Look for books that rate hostels so you know what you are getting.

While researching hostels in France, we interviewed students, backpackers, and even a group of six women who had to find a hostel because they could not find a hotel with available rooms at the last minute. Hostels typically do not take reservations, especially during their busy season when they have no problems filling beds. This can be convenient, especially if you are looking for last-minute accommodations; however, you must usually check in early in the day to get a room. The experiences were varied in the assessment of safety and cleanliness from the group we interviewed. Experiences ranged from filthy rooms to clean, well-run properties that catered to their guests. Overwhelmingly, the response was, "Know what you are getting by carrying a list of recommended hostels with you."

Also note that, because a hostel has a great website and promises that it is clean and safe, this is not necessarily a guarantee that this is what you will find. The best assurance is talking to someone who has stayed there or getting a recommendation from a respected source such as hostel guides that rate each property.

According to Tayee, a manager at the Blue Planet Hostel in Paris, hostels in France have certain government rules that must be followed, such as no loud noise, no alcohol, no hanging clothes from the windows to dry, and closing the lobby area at midnight. The Blue Planet has an attendant at the front desk at all times and locks the front door at midnight. They do not have a curfew, but the front desk attendant must check you in before entering after midnight. Keys are left at the front desk when you leave for the day, and each key is daily re-programmed to fit the electronic locks of the rooms. They also have a surveillance camera in the luggage storage room.

Most hostels will have strict hours in which you may access your room. Typically, they will close off rooms from about 11:00am –3:00pm when they will clean the rooms and bathrooms. If you check in during these times, you can leave your bags in a room provided for luggage storage, however, keep in mind that this may not be secure so take your valuables with you. There may also be an evening curfew, so know the rules before planning a late night out.

4

Finances, Phone Cards, & Travel Documents

There are many forms of currency available for today's traveler, such as U.S. cash, credit cards, traveler's checks, ATM cards and foreign currency. While planning your itinerary, budget your finances as well as your time. Estimate costs of transportation, lodging, meals, shopping, tour costs, tips—and don't forget taxes! Decide how you will pay for each of these expenses: Is lodging going to be paid by credit card? Will you need cash for taxi service, tips, and tours? Keep in mind you will want a certain amount of local currency on hand when you arrive. Be diversified. Don't count on one form of currency to meet all your needs while traveling. For safety, it is wise to take precautions and plan for emergencies.

Catherine and Debbie lingered over a sumptuous breakfast as the morning sun warmed the dining room of the quaint inn. It was a beautiful fall day in Nottingham, England, and, as they savored the last of the scones, they reviewed their itinerary, looking forward to what the day would bring. They had driven up from London the day before, chatting non-stop about the treasures they had found at the antiques market, the wild ride on the Big Red Bus, tea at The Brown's, and Debbie's first glimpse of a DaVinci in the National Gallery of Art. They had greatly anticipated their trip to Great Britain and had carefully planned an itinerary that would take them to England, Scotland, and Ireland, while allowing time for impromptu side trips should the mood strike.

Now they had a new mission: to find the famous Nottingham lace! They grabbed their new silk scarves, the one extravagant purchase from Harrod's, and walked to the lobby to pay the bill for their night's stay.

"I'm sorry Mrs. Comer, there has been a hold placed on your credit card," the innkeeper said as he stood holding the phone. " I am trying to reach the bank for you."

Catherine could not believe it! She had planned carefully to have a credit card with a limit high enough to appease her shopping goals. "I've used this credit card all over London for the past week," she cried "I know the card is good!"

The innkeeper shook his head as he replaced the phone in its cradle. "I am sorry, they have asked you to contact the fraud department of your bank."

Catherine and Debbie looked at each other, fighting the urge to panic. What about the rest of their vacation? How would they pay for their expenses? Catherine realized she had brought her debit card with her, and they had cash in their money belts. They came up with enough British pounds to pay the bill and loaded their luggage in the rental car. They left the inn with certainty that they would call the bank from the nearest pay phone and get the matter straightened out quickly.

Two days later, Catherine was finally on the phone with her bank! She now understood that the fraud department was located in the central part of the United States, in the mountain time zone, that her long distance phone card would not allow her to connect to a toll-free number in the U.S., and that the credit card company had noticed sudden international activity on her card and had placed a flag on her account, requiring identification to be checked to complete a transaction. Unfortunately, the message, which came through the banking system, was to place a hold on the account.

Could this happen to you? Even with careful planning, unforeseen incidents can occur. Understanding how and when you can use your chosen form of payment will help you to be prepared should you have problems.

Paying for Your Trip

Credit Cards

Many credit cards are widely accepted around the world. Before you leave on your trip, notify your credit card company that you will be using your card away from home. You will not usually need to notify them if you are simply traveling to another state; however, this can be critical if you are traveling internationally. Sudden use in a foreign country can "flag" attention and cause the company to place a hold on your card until they can verify that it is you who is using it. Notification can be accomplished with a simple phone call to the customer service department of your credit card company. Also ask your customer service representative what restrictions may apply and what your spending limit is.

In addition to being convenient, credit cards usually offer the best exchange rate when traveling internationally. Your credit card company will convert the amount of purchase into U.S. dollars and this will appear on your statement. You should always know the exchange rate when making a purchase so that you know what to expect on the bill when you return home.

Another benefit of using credit cards for travel expenses is that many companies offer various forms of travel insurance when purchases are made using their card. According to U.S. Bank representatives, "The level of insurance coverage Visa offers travel/emergency services is determined by the type of Visa card used. Cardholders should review the features of their card agreement and call the Visa Assistance Center if they have questions. Most Visa cards offer travel and accident insurance, auto rental insurance, and various other travel/emergency services that assist you before, during, and after your overseas travel." For example, purchasing your airline ticket with your U.S. Bank Visa® card provides you with travel accident insurance at no additional charge. American Express® is one of the largest card issuers in the world and offers extensive services for managing your finances while traveling. You can find more information about American Express's services by looking through their website at *www.americanexpress.com*. MasterCard® and other credit cards have similar benefits, so check with your provider before you travel.

Tips for choosing currency:

◆ Be diversified— use several forms such as credit card, ATM card, and cash, both in U.S. dollars and local currency

◆ Take small amounts of cash for tips, transportation, etc., when you arrive

◆ Know how to replace a credit card should it become lost or stolen

While credit cards are probably the most convenient form of payment, there are many major tourist attractions that still do not accept credit cards for entry, such as the Eiffel Tower in Paris. At sites such as these, you will need cash to buy entry tickets.

Here are some questions to ask the credit card customer service representative when calling:

- Can I use this card in _____country?
- What is my spending limit?
- What insurance benefits are provided with my credit card membership? (Lost or broken items, rental car accidents, life insurance, etc.?)
- How can I contact you if I lose my card?
- Get a local number as well as a toll-free number.
- If my card is lost or stolen, can you issue me another card immediately and where can I get it?

This information should be kept in your travel file; however, don't forget to take copies of your card numbers with you in case of an emergency. List the card numbers and phone numbers on a small card to carry in your money belt.

Cash

You will most likely need to have a small amount of cash available for expenses such as taxis, subways, small food purchases, etc. Before leaving on your trip, review your itinerary and estimate how much cash you will need for at least the first 48 hours of your trip. If you are traveling internationally, it is a good idea to have currency converted to the form of currency in the country or countries in which you will be traveling. You can go to a major branch of most banks before departure or to currency exchange bureaus at the airport of the country in which you arrive. The exchange rate will usually be better in the host country.

When traveling internationally, we recommend carrying a small, inexpensive currency converter. These resemble a small calculator and can be found at luggage and travel stores. When you are making a transaction or searching for currency exchange rates, the currency converter will allow you to enter a rate and quickly convert from foreign currency to U.S. dollars or vice versa. Even if traveling to several countries, you can easily enter the rate for that country. Have the converter handy while shopping, eating out, or making currency transactions. Keep in mind that you cannot convert change, so be sure to spend your coins in each country before leaving.

Using Automatic Teller Machines

ATMs (Automatic Teller Machines) are now very common in most cities around the world and are becoming a popular source of accessing cash while traveling. If you are using a Visa ATM card, you can access the Visa ATM locator online at *www.visa.com/pd/atm* before you go. This will provide a list of ATMs in cities around the world. MasterCard® users can log on to *www.mastercard.com/atm/* to locate ATMs throughout the U.S. and worldwide. Carrying an ATM card will allow you to carry only a small amount of cash at a time, but you will need to take care in protecting your card while you are using ATM machines. Make sure that no one standing around you can see you enter your PIN (personal identification number). There may also be a problem accessing your account from ATMs in some countries. Call your provider before leaving on your trip and ask whether your account can be accessed from a foreign country and what withdrawal limits may apply. Many international ATMs will allow you to access only your primary account, such as checking, so if you have funds in a savings account, transfer these before you leave. Have an alternative method of getting cash should your card not work. If you have problems with the ATM machine, go into a bank to access funds from your account.

Carol Rossman, group product manager for U.S. Bank, recommends being diversified when choosing travel finances. She uses credit cards, debit cards, and cash. "I do carry two cards, from two different issuers. If one is having trouble authorizing transactions or I have reached my limit on one card, I have my spare. I always use my ATM (debit card) and never have problems. I usually carry at least $100 in cash at all times. I split it up so it is not all in my purse in case I get pickpocketed."

Travelers Checks

Travelers checks can be a safe alternative to carrying cash because you can cash these on the spot and they are insured in case of loss or theft. American Express® Travelers Checks can be replaced in countries around the world, usually within 24 hours. Representatives from American Express advise taking travelers checks in local currency where possible, as most merchants will not accept them in non-local currency. If local currency travelers checks are not available, take plenty of $50 and $100 in U.S. denominations because you will usually pay a fee to cash travelers checks and using smaller denominations can be expensive and troublesome. American Express representatives told us, "You can cash American Express Travelers Cheques free of charge at any American Express office or at a network of over 65,000 other financial institutions worldwide." (See American Express for details.) You will need to show identification each time you cash a travelers check. You may receive a better exchange rate than using cash in some locations; however, consider the fees and determine what form of currency will provide the best exchange and convenience overall.

Keeping in Touch While Traveling

Making Phone Calls While Traveling

For women travelers, it can bring peace of mind to know that you can make calls in case of emergencies, contact loved ones at home, or keep up on business calls while away from home. Phone companies now offer many convenient ways to keep in touch while traveling. Types of service and charges vary greatly, so make sure you understand service options and all charges before you go. With technology constantly improving, keeping in touch while traveling is getting easier every day.

Phone Credit Cards: With a phone credit card, you can call home from almost anywhere in the world. Because it is a credit card, you will be billed for the charges, eliminating the need to carry money for phone calls. Phone charges will vary greatly and there will be additional charges such as access fees added on to the long-distance charges. Hotels will usually charge you a fee just for using the phone, whether it is a local call or a long-distance connection. Also, keep in mind that not all phone cards work at all locations, even within the U.S. For example, it may be difficult to use your phone card from your hotel room because the hotel may have a different provider, which may not be compatible. If this happens, try using a public phone to make long-distance calls, especially when calling out of the country.

When traveling internationally, call your long-distance provider before leaving on your trip to receive a list of access numbers for international calls. You will usually have to dial the access number first, then enter the number you are dialing, followed by your phone card number. This process may be reversed, depending on your provider. When placing a call, you will be given directions on the phone. Some pay phones require that you deposit a coin first before you can call the access number. The coin will be returned once the call goes through. Other phones may not require a coin at all. You can simply call the access number when you hear the dial tone. Before you go, check what rates and extra charges will apply for international calls. Some phone companies can charge up to $7 per minute for international calls.

Pre-Paid Phone Cards: A pre-paid phone card may be a less expensive alternative to the standard phone credit card. Pre-paid phone cards represent telephone time you buy in advance. You pay from $5 to $15 or more up-front for local or long-distance phone time; the amount of time you buy depends on the rate-per-minute you're charged. For many people, pre-paid phone calls offer the ultimate in convenience. The time has been paid for in advance, the card can be used from most phones, and there's no need to think about carrying coins or paying a bill later on. They come with international calling directions and an international code list. Pre-paid phone cards, which can end up costing much less than using your phone credit card, are sold at newsstands, post offices, travel agencies, retail stores, and grocery and convenience stores. They are used mostly by travelers, students, people who regularly call overseas, and those who may not have long-distance telephone service. Some pre-paid phone cards can be recharged, usually by billing the additional cost to your credit card.

Cell Phones: Cell phones are increasingly popular for keeping in touch while traveling. The benefit of cell phones is that they are small, can fit in your purse or pocket, and offer the safety and convenience of having phone service with you at all times. This can bring peace of mind for women travelers. Another plus is that you may already have a cell phone and a service plan, eliminating the need to have additional phone service charges when traveling domestically. If you have a service plan that does not include long distance, you can have this added. Check with your service provider about plans that include free long distance. Using a cell phone without the free long-distance service can result in high costs of roaming and long-distance charges. The downside to cell phones for travelers is that most do not offer service out of the country. Check with your provider and look at all charges involved.

Renting Cell Phones: You can now rent a cell phone for your next trip out of town or out of the country. You can go online to providers such as *www.worldroom.com* and rent cell phones by the week or month. The downside to this is that these are very expensive. Weekly rental costs could be approximately $70 for the use of the phone, $20 to have the phone sent to you and $30 for insurance. The price varies depending upon where you are traveling to and the service plan you want to use. Cell phones operate by satellite and are becoming increasingly popular.

Other Electronic Communication

Electronic communication is almost growing more rapidly than reports can keep up with. There are other forms of keeping in touch with loved ones at home while traveling or for communicating in case of emergencies.

WyndTell is a company that offers wireless communication for people who are hearing impaired. Operating on a compact pager, WyndTell service provides complete wireless communication via email, TTY, fax, alphanumeric paging, and even voice telephones. You can contact them for more information:

> Wynd Communications Corporation
> 75 Higuera Street, Suite 240
> San Luis Obispo, CA 93401
> Voice: 800-549-2800
> TTY: 800-549-2800
> FAX: 805-781-6001
> Website: *www.wynd.com*

Another company providing two-way interactive pagers for popular use is Motorola. Their website is *www.motorola.com*. Click on "Consumer Products."

A PDA (Personal Digital Assistant) is a handheld device that combines computing, telephone, fax, and networking. A typical PDA can function as a cellular phone, fax sender, and personal organizer. Just go to your search engine and type in PDA, and you will pull up several sites.

Email Access

Email access has grown tremendously around the world, and many hotels now offer it to their guests. Some foreign countries have Internet access businesses where you can go online for a small fee. Email providers such as Hotmail® make it easy to keep in touch with home. We both use our Hotmail® accounts while traveling internationally. It is easy to access our accounts and is more convenient than trying to schedule our phone calls to coincide with the time difference at home. *HerMail.com* is another great email provider. You can sign up for a free account and receive messages on the Internet around the world.

There are challenges with finding email access when traveling, however. Not every hotel, business, or other establishment has the latest technology to make email access feasible. Many hotels will use an older computer for Internet access for their guests. This can mean very slow connection and transport time when trying to send or download messages or information. When traveling to Mexico recently, Catherine called the hotel in Puerto Vallarta to ask if they have email access, and they said yes, it was available in the management office. What they did not say was that the computer they use for guest Internet access was older (therefore, very slow), there was a $5.80 charge just to connect, and then you had to type in a password everytime you clicked the mouse. The use of their system was so frustrating that Catherine finally gave up after the first two emails she sent.

Email Access at Hotels: If you require email access when traveling, contact the hotel before you go and ask what type of system they have in place. You will usually find more up-to-date equipment if the hotel has a business center designed with services for their guests. Connection fees will most likely depend on the type of service they have. Larger cities will have local access numbers, while smaller towns and villages may have to dial long distance to get access. They will pass this cost on to you, so ask if there is a charge to connect and if there are per-minute charges. Also ask how many terminals they have. You could end up waiting for hours if there is only one computer and many guests want to use the service.

Cyber Cafés: Cyber cafes are very popular in many parts of the world. These are centers which provide Internet services for browsing purposes at a minimum charge. We have used cyber cafes in many foreign destinations and found them to be easy to access and reasonably priced. In Paris, we accessed the Internet for one hour for about $3.00; however, you could be charged up to $12 per hour or more. Ask up-front what the charges will be. There can also be additional charges if you want to download and print information.

Modem Access

Many businesswomen travelers take their laptop computer or "notebook" with them when taking a trip. Modem access can be a challenge if not prepared. Before you go, make sure you understand how to hook your system up to a remote phone system. While you may be able to hook your computer up to the phone line in many new domestic hotels, this could be a challenge when traveling internationally. We recommend logging on to Steve Kropla's Internet site *www.kropla.com/ phones.htm*. This comprehensive guide takes you through some typical issues that may arise when hooking your modem up in a foreign country.

Travel Documents

Passports

When traveling internationally, you will need a passport. You can apply for a passport at over 4,500 passport acceptance facilities nationwide, including many post offices, some libraries, and a number of county and municipal offices. You can find a list of these facilities, by calling the National Passport Information Center at 1-900-225-5674, or you can download the form from the Internet at *www.travel.state.gov/*. Directions for applying are listed on the passport form. You should allow at least six weeks to receive your passport after it has been accepted. If you are leaving on an emergency trip, apply in person at the nearest passport agency. You must present your airline tickets or airline-generated itinerary, as well as other required items, which you can obtain by calling the agency. Many passport agencies are now operating by appointments and will serve only those leaving in less than 14-21 days.

Take a photocopy of the identification page of your passport with you when you travel, and leave a copy at home in your travel file. Don't forget to fill out your address and emergency contact information form on page five of your passport. This information can be critical if authorities need to contact a loved one at home in case you have an emergency while traveling. (Look for tips on keeping your passport safe while traveling in Chapter Eight, "Your Personal Safety Guide.")

Visas

If you are traveling to a country that requires a visa, you must obtain the visa from the embassy or consulate of the country you are planning to visit. The booklet *Foreign Entry Requirements* has information on visa/entry requirements, embassy and consulate addresses, and telephone numbers. You can obtain this booklet and additional information by visiting the State Department Internet site *www.travel.state.gov/* or by calling 202-663-1225. You can also access the website *www.embassy.org* for a list of foreign embassies that are located in the U.S. There are different kinds of visas such as those for visitors, students, immigrants and workers. Many countries will only require visas if you are planning to be in that country for an extended period of time such as traveling as a student.

Preparing for Customs and Immigration

When traveling internationally, you must go through U.S. Immigration and Customs checkpoints when returning home. This can sometime be a daunting process if you are not prepared with the proper paperwork, receipts, etc. When re-entering the U.S. by plane or cruise ship, the flight attendants or cabin stewards will hand out necessary forms for you to fill out before you disembark. You will need to present these to Immigration and Customs agents upon arrival.

Immigration

The Immigration and Naturalization Service (INS) is responsible for ensuring that individuals entering the U.S. by land, sea, or air are eligible to do so under U.S. immigration law. Travelers re-entering the U.S. will be directed through a checkpoint for verification of admissibility. If you are a frequent international traveler, you may want to contact the INS to find out about a new automated system called the Passenger Accelerated Service System (INSPASS) that can significantly reduce immigration inspection processing time for authorized travelers. You can contact the INS for specific questions at 1-800-375-5283, or access their website at *www.ins.usdoj.gov/.*

U.S. Customs

When re-entering the U.S., you will need to declare everything you brought back that you did not take with you when you left. If you are traveling by air or sea, you may be asked to fill out a Customs declaration form. The airline or cruise ship almost always provides this form.

Agents whom we interviewed at the U.S. Customs headquarters in Washington D.C., offered the following tips to make clearing Customs easier and faster:

- Know what items must be declared.

- Keep your sales slips when making purchases. Write a note on the receipt stating what the item is.

- Don't travel with expensive jewelry.

- Pack together any items that you need to declare, and, if possible, keep these separated from your other luggage. You can place these in a carry-on or in checked bags in a separate area in case you need to access the items for inspection.

- Be yourself, and answer questions honestly.

- Be aware that under U.S. law, Customs inspectors are authorized to examine luggage, cargo, and travelers.

- Contact U.S. Customs before you go if you have questions.

- Read the signs in the Customs area upon re-entry, as they contain helpful information about how to clear Customs.

Generally, items that must be declared are items you purchased, gifts you received, items you bought in duty-free shops, and items you are bringing home for someone else.

You must state on the Customs declaration, in United States currency, what you actually paid for each item, including all taxes. If the item is a gift that you received while you were in another country, you must estimate its value. You are generally allowed an exemption of $400 per person, and family members may combine their exemptions. Children and infants are allowed the same exemption as adults, except for alcoholic beverages.

Traveling with valuables: The advice from Customs agents is *don't* travel with valuables such as expensive jewelry; however, if you need to take valuables with you, register them with Customs before you go. You can register certain items with Customs before you depart, including jewelry, watches, cameras, and laptop computers, as long as they have serial numbers or other unique, permanent markings. Take the items to the nearest Customs Office and request a Certificate of Registration. You can access the U.S. Customs website listed below for an office near you, or request a registration certificate at the airport Customs office upon departure. Remember to schedule enough time to fill out forms before catching your flight.

If you have questions about what must be declared, contact U.S. Customs by calling 1-800-BE ALERT, access their website at *www.customs.gov/travel/travel.htm*, or write to the Director, Passenger Programs, U.S. Customs Service, 1300 Pennsylvania Ave. NW, Washington, D.C 20229. Their brochure, *Know Before You Go*, is an excellent resource for international travelers. You can access the information in the brochure on the Internet or request a hard copy.

Trip Insurance

When searching for trip insurance, be sure to read the brochure to determine what types of coverage is being offered. You will usually find three types of insurance: Baggage, Medical, and Cancellation.

Baggage Insurance

Baggage insurance will cover costs of lost baggage and items in the bag and can also cover costs of purchasing items in case your baggage is delayed. Airlines have guidelines for replacing lost luggage, and you may be disappointed in the amount they are willing to pay. Baggage insurance can help recover the cost of items above and beyond what the airline will reimburse you for; however, our advice is to avoid placing valuable items in checked bags. You should also check with your homeowner's insurance policy to see if baggage or lost items may be covered.

Medical and Evacuation Insurance

We discuss medical insurance in Chapter Five, "Staying Healthy while Traveling"; however, note that you can purchase traveler's health insurance on many standard travel insurance policies. Medical insurance in which the amount of coverage will depend on the type of policy you purchase and what you want covered. You can pay anywhere from $5 to $175 or more for extra medical coverage while traveling. It is important to read the benefits of the policies. Evacuation insurance can be critical to have if you need to return home unexpectedly.

Trip Cancellation/Interruption Insurance

Just as medical insurance can help cover expenses in case of accidents or illness, trip insurance can be valuable if you have to unexpectedly cancel your travel plans or come home early. For example, if you spend $5,000 booking a trip to Europe and break your leg two days before going, chances are slim that you would receive all of your money back. While you may be able to get a refund on a portion of what you paid, you will most likely have to forfeit some of the costs. Trip insurance can help recover the pre-paid travel expenses and is relatively inexpensive in comparison to the cost of an international trip.

Most professionals recommend taking out trip insurance. A good rule to follow is to determine what your travel investment is and the impact it would make if you lost that investment. Trip insurance can be purchased through your travel agent or at a variety of online resources listed below. It is important that you read the fine print and know what is covered. For example, if booking a tour or a cruise, you may think that your trip cancellation insurance will cover costs if your traveling companion becomes ill and you have to cancel. However, "traveling companion" will most likely mean one person who is booked to share the same room accommodations as you and not a traveling companion booked in a separate room. If you have to cancel because your travel companion cannot go, and she is booked in a different room, you may not get your money back.

Other Travel Insurance

What if you break a valuable piece of Venetian glass while transporting it home on the plane or the Chinese jade necklace you had shipped to Aunt Ruth while in Beijing never makes it to her door?

There are a variety of insurance policies that can help. If you purchased your Venetian glass with your credit card, it may be insured through your card provider. Check before you travel to find out what insurance benefits are available on credit cards and on homeowners insurance and trip insurance policies. It can make a difference in the event that something happens to your valuables while traveling. American Express, Visa, MasterCard, and other credit card providers have policies regarding replacement of lost or broken items purchased with the credit card. Check with your credit card company before traveling to find out what types of insurance benefits apply. Knowing the benefits ahead of time can help you determine which method you should use in purchasing items while traveling, especially valuable items.

Insurance Resources

- **Travel Agents or Tour Company:** Ask your travel agent or tour coordinator to recommend a travel insurance provider. They will provide you with brochures and applications and will handle the insurance purchase for you.

- **Credit Card Provider:** Check with your credit card company for insurance benefits included with your card

- **Homeowners Insurance:** Check your policy to see if lost luggage and other items may be covered

- **Travel Insurance Providers:** These are companies that provide different types of insurance for travelers. Read all policies carefully before purchasing

World Travel Center—
www.worldtravelcenter.com
1-800-786-5566 or +1 (402) 397-3311; ask for travel dept.
(7:30 to 5:00 M-Th and 7:30-2:30 F CST USA)

Council Travel—
www.counciltravel.com/travelinsurance
They have policies for student and budget travelers.

Global Travel Insurance—
www.globaltravelinsurance.com
You can get an online quote here.

CSA Travel protection—
www.csatravelprotection.com/insure/tr_order.asp

5

Staying Healthy While Traveling

Preparing for a healthy trip is as important as researching your destination, choosing safe transportation and lodging, and organizing your packing. Planning a trip with health in mind is a matter of reviewing your destination and itinerary and considering ways to stay healthy while traveling.

A great resource for planning travel with health in mind is Medicine Planet. Their website, *www.medicineplanet.com,* not only offers travel planning advice, but also includes a list of travel clinics located throughout the U.S.

Ricki Pollycove, MD, MHS is a nationally recognized expert on a broad range of issues pertaining to the traveling woman. Dr. Pollycove recommends a routine check-up with your doctor prior to traveling, especially if planning to be away from home for longer than two weeks. She recommends that her patients take preventive medications for problems such as bladder and yeast infections, traveler's diarrhea, jet lag, and motion sickness. Her overriding theme for advice to women who travel is to drink plenty of water. "Dehydration is one of the biggest problems travelers face because it affects our bodies in a variety of ways. It makes us more susceptible to swelling, bladder infections, and even more serious ailments because without proper hydration, we do not get rid of the toxins in our systems. Contrary to what some people think, drinking more water will actually help reduce swelling because it will flush the salt out as well." She suggests carrying bottled water with you at all times wherever you are traveling.

Dr. Pollycove's top tips:

- Have a routine check-up with your doctor.
- Take extra medications.
- Drink plenty of bottled water.
- Wear support stockings such as support panty hose or support tights.
- *Never* wear knee high socks when traveling unless they are made by a support hose company such as Jobst. (You can access their website at *www.jobst-usa.com/*, call 419-698-1611, or write to them at Jobst, 653 Miami St., Toledo, OH 43605 to find a retailer near you).
- Avoid ankle socks that have a constrictive band.
- Place a blanket across your lap and feet while on a plane to keep your joints warm and improve circulation.
- Flex your feet and point your toes every two hours.

Another resource is the International Association for Medication Assistance to Travellers (IAMAT). They provide a contact list of English-speaking doctors located around the world. This could be invaluable if you are traveling with a medical condition. You can call them at 716-754-4883 or access their website at *www.sentex.net/~iamat.*

Get plenty of rest before taking a trip and practice healthy eating habits. Make sure that you have had your annual check-up with your doctor. If you have a high-risk medical condition, consult your doctor before traveling. Ask your physician what precautions you may need to take, as well as what medications or special equipment you will need to pack.

Recent studies indicate that it is advisable to eat and drink something healthy before flying. Many of us assume that we can eat on the plane, especially when taking early morning flights; however, it is easy to misjudge the time when you may actually get your meal. For example, if you get up at 5:00am for an 8:00am flight, you may think that you will eat on the plane and be tempted to skip breakfast at home. In reality, by the time the plane boards, takes off, and arrives at a cruising altitude safe for serving meals, it may be close to 10:00am before you actually receive something to eat or drink.

If you require a special diet, be sure to let the agent who books the ticket or the airline know in advance of your departure day, and they will mark this in your flight record. Whether you need a low-sodium meal or you are a vegetarian, the airlines will usually try to accommodate your request if notified beforehand.

If resting on a plane while traveling is difficult for you, think about ways to make yourself more comfortable, especially if taking long flights and you need to sleep. Ask your doctor to recommend a medication that will help you sleep. We like to take an inflatable neck pillow, as these fold flat and can be tucked into our carry-on and blown up for use.

Health habits that we take for granted at home are not necessarily safe practices in foreign countries. Lavon took great care while in Argentina to drink only bottled water; however, she brushed her teeth with tap water, thinking that she would be safe if she did not swallow. She became ill, as many people do when drinking tap water while in foreign countries. She was ill for two days. What began as a simple habit of brushing teeth, turned into two days of misery. The problem is not necessarily that there is anything wrong with the tap water in all foreign countries. The concern is that we have not developed immunities to certain organisms or parasites in the water. Again, check with your doctor for preventive medications if you are prone to problems or are traveling to foreign countries where this may be an issue.

Traveler's Illnesses

Traveler's Diarrhea

This is perhaps one of the most common ailments faced by international travelers. If you have ever suffered from traveler's diarrhea, you most likely have experienced getting on a plane with the fear that you may have to dash down the aisle to the nearest toilet. There are many remedies available for treating traveler's diarrhea. Most medications are now available in chewable tablets as well as liquid. We strongly recommend packing a supply in your first aid traveler's kit, which you will take in your carry-on luggage. Ask your doctor which medication would work best for you. Be sure to let your doctor know of any other medications you are taking and ask for possible risks of mixing drugs whether prescription or over-the-counter.

Women may especially be prone to problems because of another common condition called Irritable Bowel Syndrome (IBS). According to recent studies, two-thirds of people who suffer from IBS are women. The common symptoms of IBS are abdominal pain, diarrhea, bloating, and a change in your bowel function. A change in diet and daily routine can be a large contributor to this condition. If you suffer from IBS on a regular basis, it would be wise to consult your physician before going on a trip.

Some tips for guarding against traveler's diarrhea:

- Drink bottled water. Avoid ice in drinks.

- Brush your teeth with bottled water. (Although many hotels have a water purification system, which will make the tap water safe for drinking and brushing teeth, if you are in doubt, use bottled water.)

- Eat cooked foods—do not eat raw fruits and vegetables unless they can be peeled.

- Avoid food from street vendors.

- Ask your doctor to prescribe a medication for parasites, as this can be the cause of illness from water sources.

Don Comer, who has been a corporate traveler for 20 years, experienced the unexpected while on a business trip to Spain. "I took precautions against illness by drinking bottled water, brushing my teeth with bottled water, and not ordering ice in any drinks. What I was not prepared for was being served chilled soup during a business lunch. I assumed that the soup had been cooked before chilling but discovered too late, that the soup base was made with local tap water and had not been boiled."

Blisters and Foot Ailments

Perhaps nothing can ruin a great day of walking and exploring a travel destination quite as much as developing blisters or sore feet. You will find tips on choosing and packing comfortable shoes in Chapter Seven, "What to Pack." However, as careful as you may be in choosing shoes well, foot problems may happen. Carry padded, adhesive bandages with you in case a blister occurs. When you arrive at your hotel for the evening, rub lotion on your feet and prop them up. Remember to alternate the shoes you wear to give your feet a rest from the same fit every day.

Jet Lag and Sleep Deprivation

Many travelers suffer from jet lag, which is a sleep disorder considered to be caused by disruption of your "body clock," a small cluster of brain cells that controls the timing of biological functions (circadian rhythms), including when you eat and sleep. There are pills available to help prevent jet lag. As with any medication, check with your doctor first.

Here are some general tips to prevent jet lag:

- Select flights that will allow you to arrive at your destination early enough in the evening to settle in and get a good night's sleep before starting meetings or tours the next day.

- If you are traveling at night, try to sleep on the plane. Don't be tempted to stay up and watch the movie.

- Ear plugs and blindfolds can be very helpful in blocking out unwanted noise and light.

- Avoid alcohol and caffeine while traveling and before bedtime hours.

- Heavy meals can also alter your sleep pattern. Eat lightly and healthfully.

- Change your watch to your destination time upon boarding your plane. This will help you adjust to the time change while traveling.

- Try to stay as close as possible to your normal schedule. If possible, take travel recovery time into consideration when planning your itinerary. For example, if you have a Monday morning meeting scheduled in Paris, travel on Friday. You will arrive on Saturday because of the time change, which will leave you Sunday to rest before starting your week.

Altitude Pressure and Dry Cabin Air

Try to pop your ears as you ascend and descend. You can accomplish this by yawning or chewing gum. If you have a problem with your ears and they will not unplug, consult your physician.

The pressurized air in the cabin of the plane can be very drying. In addition to drinking plenty of water, take throat lozenges to ease dryness and hydrate your skin with a good moisturizing lotion. If you wear contacts, be sure to take re-wetting drops for your eyes.

Motion Sickness

If you are prone to motion sickness, ask your doctor to recommend a preventive medication. These are available in pills and patches.

Tips to help prevent motion sickness:

* Try to keep your head as still as possible while traveling and focus on a distant object.
* Avoid reading.
* Nibble on crackers such as saltines.

Protection from the Sun

Exposure to the sun's ultraviolet (UV) rays is an important health issue for traveling women, as reports indicate that this is the most important factor in the development of skin cancer. Your destination will play a critical role in how much exposure to these harmful rays you will have. For example, if you are traveling to the tropics, you will need more protection than traveling to northern climates; however, keep in mind that even in areas where there is not a lot of sun, ultraviolet rays can penetrate the thin atmosphere.

According to Shaun Hughes, president of Sun Precautions, Inc., "Women are smart about pursuing good health, including good skin health. However, many don't realize what a silent killer skin cancer can be. The deadliest form of skin cancer, malignant melanoma, is the number one form of terminal cancer of all kinds for women aged 25-30, and second in incidence behind breast cancer for women aged 30-35. Women's most marked place to get this form of skin cancer is on the lower leg.

Skin cancer is chiefly caused by over-exposure to the sun. Sun protection should begin at sun up and end at sun down. A minor sunburn in Miami can happen in as little as 5 minutes in the summer. So any time you're outside, you need to practice head-to-toe sun protection." Hughes's company specializes in sun protection clothing.

Many women may not be aware of other factors contributing to increased sensitivity to the sun. Perfumes, lotions, and medications such as antibiotics and estrogen are just some of the daily items used by women that may increase their skin's sensitivity to the sun. Before traveling, check with your doctor or pharmacist if taking medications. Even some over-the-counter medications can cause sun sensitivity. According to one pharmacist, "Do not rely on lists of medications (typically posted in places such as sun tanning salons) which increase sun sensitivity because there are simply too many medications to properly list warnings for all of them." A patient information sheet will accompany most prescriptions. Read this to see if

✗ ———————————

Sun Protection Tips

◆ Limit exposure to the sun, especially when traveling to the tropics.

◆ Wear lotion with a sun protection factor recommended by your doctor or dermatologist.

◆ Wear a hat.

◆ Wear lightweight clothing that protects your skin.

◆ Check with your doctor or pharmacist when taking any medications, even over-the-counter drugs that may increase your skin's sensitivity to the sun.

◆ Wear sunglasses when outside on bright days.

◆ Drink plenty of fluids.

✗

there is mention of increased sensitivity to the sun. If it is not mentioned, ask the pharmacist.

Stick with lotions that are specifically formulated for sun protection and avoid wearing perfume when in the sun.

Resources for Sun Protection Information

The National Center for Disease Control
Website: *http://www.cdc.gov/*
(Under "search," type in sun protection)
Phone: 404-639-3534 or 800-311-3435
Address: Centers for Disease Control and Prevention
1600 Clifton Rd.
Atlanta, GA 30333

Earthlink: This will take you to an article about every-day products that may make you sun sensitive.
http://home.earthlink.net/~sberkowitz/Sunburn.html

Expedia: This is a valuable travel-related website.
www.expedia.com
(Search for sun protection to find articles)

Sun Precautions®: Specialists in sun protection clothing.
Phone: 800-882-7860
www.sunprecautions.com

Traveler's Stress

Travel delays, lost luggage, jet lag, and unmet expectations are just some of the challenges that face many travelers. These situations can be very frustrating for any woman and especially women who are traveling with children and have to tend to them as well as trying to keep track of their tickets, carry-ons, etc.

Whether traveling by car, plane, or public transportation, try to relax and face each situation as it arises. In some cases, you will find that a sense of humor will help relieve the pressure.

Other Health Considerations

Prescriptions

If you require medication, take enough extra in case of extended stays. Pack your prescriptions in your carry-on luggage in case your checked bags become lost. If you have a serious medical condition that requires medication, ask your doctor to provide a copy of your prescription. Carry the copy separately from the medication itself. Make sure that it is typed or clearly written. Also, have the name and phone number of your doctor in case of emergencies.

Catherine suggests having your prescriptions filled well in advance of your trip. "I called in a refill for my hormone pills prior to a trip to Germany. When I went to pick it up the night before I left, the pharmacist told me that I was five days early for my refill. Fortunately, they were able to call the insurance company to approve the refill. However, I learned not to wait until the last minute to have prescriptions filled."

U.S. Customs representatives recommend keeping your prescriptions in the original bottle to avoid questions. Some medications are considered illegal in foreign countries. If you have a specific medical condition that requires an unusual medication or a drug you are uncertain of, consult your physician before you travel. Let him/her know your destination and ask what precautions you may need to take. You can also visit the embassy website of the country you will be visiting for listings of medications that may not be allowed in that country. For a list of medications that may not be allowed in certain countries, visit *www.customs.ustreas.gov/travel/travel.htm,* website of U.S. Customs.

Traveling with Medical Equipment

Syringes, which may be necessary for diabetics and other conditions, should be accompanied by a doctor's note in the event that you are questioned during the Customs process. Ask your doctor for a statement explaining that you need the insulin or other medications and syringes for your medical condition.

Immunizations & Health Precautions

If you are traveling to a foreign country and immunizations are required, you may need to visit a travel clinic, as not all doctors carry certain medications for travel immunizations. Indeed, many doctors are not kept aware of current immunization requirements. You will need to make an appointment in advance and also allow time for certain immunizations to take effect before traveling. Make sure that your regular vaccinations, such as tetanus, are up to date.

Information on vaccinations and other health precautions may be obtained from the Centers for Disease Control and Prevention's international traveler's hotline at 1-877-FYI-TRIP (1-877-394-8747), via their autofax service at 1-888-CDC-FAXX (1-888-232-3229), or their Internet homepage at *http:// www.cdc.gov.*

The U.S. State Department Consular Sheets will also provide a list of health problems for each country, or you can access the website of the World Health Organization: *http://www.who.int/*.

Disinsection

Aircraft disinsection is the spraying of insecticides on airplanes in certain countries. It is permitted under international law in order to protect public health, agriculture, and the environment. The World Health Organization and the International Civil Aviation Organization stipulate two approaches for aircraft disinsection: either spray the aircraft cabin with an aerosolized insecticide while passengers are on board, or treat the aircraft's interior surfaces with a residual insecticide (residual method) while passengers are *not* on board.

We have experienced this spraying upon landing in certain countries. The flight attendants came through the cabin and handed out washcloths to place over our face. They then walked through the aircraft and sprayed, using a can of insecticide. If you think you may be allergic to the process and are traveling to a country where this disinsection may occur, check with the airline before you go. You may be able to de-plane prior to spraying. You can find a list of countries that practice aircraft disinsection at *http://ostpxweb.dot.gov/policy/safety/disin.htm.*

Female Health Concerns

Monthly Cycle

If there is a possibility that you may start your period while traveling, take a supply of sanitary products. Some products may not be easily available in foreign countries. Take care to cleanse yourself well while traveling to avoid problems with infection. If you require medication for cramps, take it with you, since many medications, even over-the-counter drugs, may not be easy to find while traveling.

Bladder and Yeast Infections

Bladder and yeast infections are common for women travelers and can be caused by such factors as using dirty public toilets and dehydration. Public toilets in many foreign countries may not be the same as those you are used to at home.

Dr. Pollycove recommends:

- Drink ample purified water and other fluids.
- Consider drinking cranberry juice and taking vitamin C tablets.
- Keep your genitals clean and avoid irritants.

There is also a risk of your skin becoming irritated by the toilet paper so pack a tube of anti-itch cream. This will also come in handy for insect bites and other minor skin irritations. Ask your doctor or pharmacist for advice on which product to use.

Medical Insurance

To Buy Coverage or Not?

Check with your medical insurance provider before you travel to find out if you are covered if you need medical assistance while traveling. This can most likely be accomplished in a five-minute phone call.

Here are some questions to ask your medical insurance provider:

- Does your policy cover medical treatment in a foreign country?
- If so, what are the limits of your coverage?
- What is the procedure for filing a claim?

Medicare's booklet, *Medicare & You 2001,* states:

> "The Original Medicare Plan generally does not cover care outside the United States, but some Medicare managed care plans, private fee–for-service plans, and Medigap policies do. Check your insurance coverage before you travel outside the country."

Many insurance companies require you to pay for medical procedures at the time of treatment. Indeed, many doctors and hospitals may expect immediate payment in cash. You will then have to apply for reimbursements when you return to the U.S. Many foreign hospitals and medical clinics will accept only major credit cards as payment for treatment.

Twenty-five year veteran travel agent Shirley Reeves remembers an incident in Mexico. She was escorting a tour when one of the travelers, a young woman, needed an emergency appendectomy. Since the clinic would only perform medical treatment if the procedure were pre-paid, Shirley had to use a credit card to pay for the surgery. She recommends that her clients always purchase travelers medical insurance.

Medical evacuation is another concern while traveling, especially internationally. If you need to either return home for an emergency or require immediate emergency transport home, the costs can become astronomical. Medical evacuation can easily cost $10,000 and up, depending on your location and medical condition. Evacuation insurance is usually an option when buying travelers medical insurance.

Our best advice for travel health is to check with your doctor before traveling. Plan ahead to include necessary items to take with you and preventive procedures in case of problems. Taking the time to prepare for a healthy trip will help you enjoy your journey more.

6

Starting a Travel File

"What was the name of the hotel where we stayed?"
*"Does our insurance cover us if we get sick while
we are traveling?"*
"Are our passports up to date?"

Have you asked yourself similar questions when planning a trip? Keeping track of travel information, such as favorite places to stay, insurance coverage, etc., can not only assist you in travel planning, but it can also provide critical information should you have an emergency while traveling.

Whether you are taking a two-day trip or a three-week excursion, it is a good idea to have a travel file. This is where you will keep pertinent information such as insurance documents, medical records, passport copies, brochures, notes from previous trips, and other related material. This file should be available to your emergency contact at home in case you have problems while traveling. It will also prove invaluable for future travel planning. Much of this information you will only need to gather once and can be obtained by phone. This file can be as extensive or as brief as you wish.

Representatives of the U.S. State Department encourage travelers to have copies of pertinent information. "It makes our job easier to assist travelers when they have copies of information such as passports and emergency contact numbers." They also suggest that travelers have access to insurance and medical information records in case of emergency. Having these records available in a travel file at home can assist if an emergency arise while you are traveling, whether domestically or internationally.

We suggest that you make two copies of your critical contact names and phone numbers, your credit card numbers, and passport. Leave one copy at home in your travel file and carry the other with you in your hidden money belt while traveling. List your contact names and phone numbers on a credit card size piece of paper, allowing you to tuck it into your

Critical information to include in your travel file

◆ Insurance documents
◆ Passport copies
◆ Medical records
◆ Credit card numbers and expiration dates
◆ Itineraries
◆ Emergency contacts such as your doctor's name and phone number

Optional information to include

◆ Brochures of places you would like to go
◆ Internet resources
◆ Copies of magazine articles

money belt. If you wish, you can have it laminated for durability (this can be done usually for less than one dollar at a local printer) and carry like a credit card.

Critical Information to Include in Your Travel File

Insurance Documents

Health Insurance: Keep a copy of your insurance policy, contact phone numbers, and policy numbers. Make notes on what is covered while you are away from home. (Refer to Chapter Six, "Staying Healthy While Traveling," for more information.)

Travelers Insurance: If you use travelers insurance, keep copies of policies or brochures for quick reference. These policies can include trip interruption or cancellation insurance, travel life insurance, baggage replacement, and travel medical coverage.

Credit Card Insurance Coverage: Many credit cards will provide travel insurance for a variety of situations such as lost luggage, lost or broken items, and even life and medical coverage if your trip is paid using the card. Know what your credit card covers while traveling, and keep a copy of the policy.

Passport Copies

If you are a frequent international traveler, keep your passport up to date in case of last-minute trips, as it can sometimes take several weeks to receive or renew a passport. Some countries require that your U.S. passport be valid at least six months or longer beyond the dates of your trip. If your passport expires before the required validity, you will have to apply for a new one. (Steps for applying for or renewing a passport are covered in Chapter Four under Travel Documents.)

Make two copies of your passport, put one in your travel file, and take one with you while traveling. In the event of loss or theft, the easiest way for agents to help you replace your passport is if you have a copy with you.

Credit Card Numbers and Contacts

Write down the card number, expiration date, and contact phone numbers of all credit cards and phone cards, and also note travelers check replacement numbers. Again, have two copies, one to take with you and one to leave at home in your travel file.

Emergency Contact Names

These are phone numbers and/or email addresses of family or friends, doctors, etc. you may need to contact in case of an emergency while traveling.

Medical Records

If you have a specific health condition or especially if you have a life-threatening illness and need to travel, it is a good idea to keep records that can assist you in case of emergencies while traveling. Ask your doctor for a copy of your condition explaining what the condition is and possible treatment needs. Carry a copy of this with you when you travel, and keep a copy in your travel file at home in case you become incapable of taking care of yourself while traveling. If you become ill while traveling or need medical assistance, you can present this to the attending physician to give them a better understanding of your medical condition. If you must travel internationally with a life-threatening illness, it would be advisable to have your condition translated into the language of the country you will be visiting. Remember to carry copies in your money belt and never place them in your checked luggage.

Optional Information for Your Travel File

Brochures

Brochures of places you have been or would like to go will help you when you are ready to plan your trip. If you loved a hotel you stayed at, keep a brochure so that you will have that information if you want to return. If you see a brochure of somewhere you would like to go someday or know you will be traveling to, tuck it in your travel file for future reference.

Internet Resources

Website address lists can save hours of online searching. Keep lists of favorite travel websites (also don't forget to bookmark them on your browser if you will be using them soon).

Copies of Magazine and Newspaper Articles, and Notes

Clip articles from magazines and newspapers for future travel planning. Keep notes from friends who have shared personal recommendations of places you may want to visit.

7

Packing With Safety and Health in Mind

By understanding how to travel with safety and health in mind, each packing experience will become easier. There are certain staples you will always need when traveling away from home. We have learned to pack lightly. We have both suffered strained muscles from lifting over-stuffed suitcases and learning the hard way to cut down on unnecessary items. Even lightweight carry-on bags can become cumbersome during long layovers at airports. While on a six-hour layover from Atlanta to Zurich, we were able to store our carry-on bags in a locker, but, during a recent delay from Chicago to Paris we were forced to contend with our carry-on bags, as lockers were unavailable. Many airports have removed lockers due to security issues, therefore, they cannot be counted on if your plane is delayed and you want to walk around. Not only will traveling lighter be easier on you physically; you will tend to be safer without a lot of bags to keep track of.

Catherine is a self-admitted shopper. "After 20 years of traveling, I have learned to pack well by packing lightly and taking only what I need. However, I love to shop and I have strained more than one muscle trying to bring everything back on the plane with me! I have waddled down the plane aisle with the seams of my carry-on stretched to the limit and extra bags over each arm. On our last trip to London, my friend Debbie and I both bought extra suitcases just to carry our antique silver purchases! Then, of course, we were afraid of our bags being lost if we checked them, so we carried them on the plane with us. A week of therapy took care of the aches and pains caused by the shopping spree. I learned from this experience to ship items home instead of trying to struggle to take them on the plane. Shipped items can be insured and you do not have to worry about them while traveling, especially if going to more than one destination on a single trip. You do not want to have to pack these items every time you change hotels.

The benefit of bringing home souvenirs is that our home is filled with wonderful memories of places my husband and I have visited around the world. I have learned over the years how to pack with the idea that I will want to bring extra things home with me. I take an extra carry-on bag for small items and ship larger items home through insured mail. Remember to contact U.S. Customs for their brochure *Know Before You Go* to understand what items can be shipped back to the U.S. Call them at 1-800-BE ALERT, or access their website at *www.customs.gov/travel/travel.htm*

It is still sometimes difficult to determine what we may need when traveling, especially when thinking of personal care. My mother and I love to take road trips by car. Mom is a great packer, although I tease her about taking everything but the kitchen sink! She packs well in advance of our trip and tucks in extra comfort items that many people never think about. During one of our road trips, we were traveling through Yellowstone National Park and I had just moved Mom's purse to the back seat and noticed how heavy it was. I was teasing her about packing so much as I slid behind the wheel and started driving through the park. I started scratching my head and said that it was strange but I had developed an itchy scalp and it was driving me crazy. Without a word, Mom reached into her purse and handed me an ointment made for itchy scalps!"

Your destination and itinerary will dictate how much and what kinds of items you will need to pack.

Ask yourself these questions:

- What is the climate and temperature of my destination?
- How long will I be away from home?
- What does my itinerary include? (Will I be walking, attending business meetings, swimming, etc?)
- What necessary items will I need? (Toiletries, first-aid items, etc.)

We approach our packing by separating our items in two categories:

1. *Carry-on:* Items that are absolutely needed while traveling and cannot easily be replaced.

2. *Checked luggage:* Items that can be replaced at our destination.

Packing Lightly

Luggage

The type of clothing you will need will determine the size and amount of luggage you require. The key considerations when choosing your luggage are protecting your valuables and being able to handle your luggage with ease. Pack lightly! Choose a suitcase with rollers and collapsible handle. You may want to consider taking an extra folding bag for bringing home items such as souvenirs. Remember, you are packing with your health and personal safety in mind. Health considerations such as back injuries from lifting over-sized luggage can ruin your trip! If you decide to take your luggage onboard the airplane, take into consideration the weight when lifting to overhead bins. You may want to check larger items, but, keep in mind your valuables should never be placed in checked baggage. You will also need to be aware of airline regulations regarding luggage size for both checked and carry-on bags.

The most common color of luggage nowadays is black. Keep this in mind as you choose your bag. Mark luggage with an identifiable tag that will make it easier to spot when claiming bags at luggage carousels. A bright yellow tag, for example, will make your bag stand out from the average black ones. Identity tags should always have a cover flap so that your name and contact information are not easily read by casual observers. Use your first initial and last name and your office address and phone number if possible on luggage tags. Also don't forget to place an identification card inside your luggage should the exterior tag be torn off during handling.

Carry-On Bags

Your carry-on luggage should contain everything necessary for you to make it a day or two if your luggage gets lost. These items will include your small purse, toiletries, travel necessities, water, snacks, reading material, and your valuables. A lightweight backpack can be an ideal carry-on piece, but do not place valuable items in outside pockets or compartments. A backpack will allow your hands to be free and may be easier to manage than a shoulder bag. The weight distribution can also be easier on your back. When standing in crowds or using public transportation such as shuttles, hold your bag in front of you with zippered pockets facing in. Choose whichever carry-on works best for your needs, taking care that it cannot easily be accessed while standing in a crowded airport.

Items to Include in Your Carry-on

Small Purse: For use while out during the day, we prefer a small purse with a strap long enough to wear diagonally over your torso. Keep only the funds you will need for the day. You can usually fit other small items such as lip protection and sunglasses in as well.

First Aid Kit: See what to include listed below.

Bottle of Water: Choose plastic bottles, as these are lighter—you can usually buy bottled water at your destination and will only need to take enough for your actual travel time until you can purchase more at your destination.

Snacks: Protein bars, granola, etc.

✈
First Aid Travel Kit

- Adhesive bandages in various sizes
- Ointments such as antibiotic ointment, anti-itching cream, and insect repellent
- Diarrhea treatment medication
- Anti-bacterial towelettes or liquid hand sanitizer
- Antacid pills
- Sunblock cream

✈

Prescriptions: Have your pharmacist fill your prescriptions for the length of stay and include enough extra for emergency bottles.

Toiletries Kit: See what to include listed below.

Reading Material: Choose paperbacks, as they are lighter.

Pen: Especially if traveling internationally, you will need to fill out immigration and Customs forms on the plane or ship.

Inflatable Neck Pillow: These will fold flat.

Folding Umbrella: This will be handy if arriving in rainy climates.

First Aid Travel Kit

You will want to build a first aid kit that will include those necessary items needed in case of minor discomfort such as traveler's diarrhea, blisters, heartburn, etc. Keep this stocked and ready to go, but check expiration dates on items regularly. You will add to the basic items depending on your personal health needs. If you are allergic to bees, for example, an emergency anti-bee sting kit may be necessary.

While on a recent trip to Seoul, Catherine and Don were forced to search for bandages and peroxide for an infected incision on Don's arm. This proved difficult, as the drugstores in Seoul are not stocked with the same items as in the U.S., and language was a barrier.

Carry-on Toiletries Kit

Your carry-on toiletries kit should be small, lightweight, and contain items necessary while traveling and in case your luggage is lost. These will include toothbrush, toothpaste, sunscreen, contact lens supplies, etc. Items such as shampoo and a sewing kit, may be packed in your checked baggage, as these items are more easily replaced if your luggage is lost. Many hotels provide these necessary items for guests. Items such as contact lens solution can be purchased in small travel-size bottles.

Carry-on Toiletries Kit

- Toothbrush, toothpaste, & dental floss
- Hairbrush
- Contact lens supplies
- Deodorant
- Spare eyeglasses
- Sunglasses
- Hand lotion
- Make-up kit
- Mouthwash
- Tissues
- Small scissors

There are toiletries or cosmetic bags available in which you can pack all your items, including first aid supplies, in one convenient bag. Many bags come with small bottles for shampoo, conditioner, etc. We have both found cosmetic bags that will accommodate all of our toiletries and first aid supplies and yet are small, lightweight, and convenient to place in our carry-on luggage. We keep these stocked and ready to travel. Take care to check expiration dates on certain items such as medications.

Money Belt and Purses

We strongly urge you to buy a personal money belt, such as a lightweight fabric pouch with elastic to fit around your waist or a fabric purse that hangs around your neck that you wear under your shirt. This is worn under your clothing and should not be detectable by passersby. As previously discussed, this will hold emergency currency and credit cards, etc. Loose-fitting clothing will allow you to conceal your money belt as well as provide access when necessary. Remember, you will need your passport and travel documents in an easily accessed place such as your carry-on while en route; however, once you arrive at your destination, place these in your money belt. These are critical items to keep on your person at all times to help prevent theft and to access in case of emergency.

What to Take in Your Money Belt

- ◆ Passport (once you arrive at your destination)
- ◆ Extra credit card
- ◆ Copy of itinerary
- ◆ Driver's license
- ◆ Emergency phone numbers
- ◆ Contact at home
- ◆ Consulate or embassy phone numbers
- ◆ Health insurance card and phone numbers
- ◆ Phone card
- ◆ Currency (include U.S. currency as well as host country)

As we stated, we recommend that purses be small, lightweight, and used for items you will need for the day such as one credit card, a small amount of cash, sun protection, a small bottle of water, and sunglasses. Keep other valuables such as extra cash and credit cards in your money belt.

Remember to keep your purse zipped with pockets facing your body when not in use. While on a water-taxi in Venice,

Catherine's sister-in-law Phyllis watched as a man reached into a friend's purse. Phyllis immediately grabbed the purse and moved her friend out of the man's way.

Clothing

With today's fabric choices and shoe designs, you do not need to sacrifice fashion for comfort. Learning how to layer your clothing will allow comfortable travel in many climates. While you may like to take your entire wardrobe with you (and many have tried), we recommend packing lightly. Choose loose-fitting clothing in layers that can be mixed and matched for a variety of looks. Loose-fitting clothing is especially important when traveling on international flights, as your legs and feet tend to swell. We prefer separates in a knit fabric that does not wrinkle easily. Pants with an elastic waist are comfortable for sitting for long periods of time on planes or in cars. For buisness travel, the "little black dress" in a knit is a versatile choice. You can wear it with a blazer, dress it up with pearls, or dress it down with flats. The look is timeless, understated, and almost always fitting. There are companies which specialize in travel clothing. You can find comfortable ensembles in a variety of styles to fit your travel agenda. Another benefit to these new knit blends is that they can be rolled to fit in your suitcase and shaken out to wear. The mix-and-match designs, besides being versatile for wearing, will also require less packing, making your luggage lighter in weight.

Avoid clothing with outside pockets, as you may be inclined to place items or money in pockets when hurrying through purchases. Expert pickpockets can get into pockets and purses you may think are secured.

Take care in choosing clothing styles appropriate to your destination (your destination research should help you make wise clothing choices). Many foreign countries are conservative in women's apparel; for example, shorts and sleeveless tops are unacceptable while touring most cathedrals in Europe. If the day is hot, wrap a lightweight sweater over your shoulders and slip it on when entering a religious facility. Most do not require a covered head, but having a small scarf tucked in your purse will come in handy if you get into this situation. A good alternative to shorts is to wear a lightweight skirt or dress.

 A pair of jeans, T-shirt, and tennis shoes can be a sure sign of a tourist. If you are traveling with a large group in a tour, you may be okay with this type of dress, but, if you are alone, you could stand out. Dark colors and conservative styles are the most preferred choices. Remember, your goal is your safety. Do not draw attention to yourself and be targeted as a tourist. A lightweight jacket or coat is advisable in case of weather changes. We love the new microfiber coats that can be folded up to fit in a pouch, although we have never actually been able to get them comfortably back into their pouch. They do however, fold up to a small size and can be shaken out quickly to wear over either business or leisure outfits. A hat can come in handy for protecting you from sun or rain.

Several of the companies that specialize in travel clothing are:

- Travel Smith (*www.travelsmith.com*) is one of the most visible providers of travel clothing and accessories because they have a magazine that you can subscribe to and they advertise in most in-flight publications.

- Changes in Latitude (*www.cil.com*) Like Travel Smith, this is a full-service on-line travel store with clothing as one of their many offerings.
- Weekenders (*www.weekenders.com*) A direct-sell company. You will need to find the local area representative by accessing their website providing your address and waiting for them to email you back with a local contact.

Jewelry

Leave your valuable jewelry at home. If your itinerary requires formal attire, take jewelry that can be placed in a small jewelry pouch that you can keep with you or leave in the hotel safety deposit box.

Shoes and Socks

As you plan your trip, consider how much walking you will be doing; for example, a lot of walking for sightseeing, or going back and forth to meetings. Pack at least two pairs of comfortable shoes. Don't be tempted to sacrifice comfort for fashion while traveling. No matter how good a shoe looks, *you* will not look great if you are hobbling along in pain. With today's variety of styles, you can have both; however, given the choice, opt for comfort. Slip-on shoes are great for wearing on the plane as they can easily be slipped off, allowing you to flex your muscles and get your blood circulating. Remember, that feet tend to swell on planes and your footwear should allow for this. Tuck a pair of socks into your carry-on bag in case your feet get cold, but take care that they do not bind around your legs. Socks should be loose fitting around your ankles unless they are support stockings made specifically for traveling. (See Chapter Five on health tips for buying stockings.) If you buy new shoes for your trip, wear them at home and *slightly* break them in before packing them. Breaking shoes in too much actually breaks down the support, which could cause problems if you need to do a lot of walking.

Hair Dryers, Curling Irons, and Converter Kits

Most domestic hotels and many international hotels provide hair dryers in their guestrooms. Ask when making reservations whether one is provided. Keep in mind that if you bring your own hair dryer, you may not be able to use it, as many bathroom outlets will only allow electric shavers, especially those in foreign countries. If traveling internationally, you will need an electrical converter kit. Whereas in the U.S. we use 110-volt alternating current, most other countries use 220-volt alternating current. Converter kits are available at travel stores and some variety stores. These will have directions with appropriate plugs for electrical outlets in various countries. If you use a curling iron, another alternative is to purchase a butane curling iron, also available at variety stores. Access Steve Kropla's website at *http://www.kropla.com/* for information about electricity around the world and what adapters will be needed to access plug-ins.

Other Items

Other items you may need will depend on your destination, type of travel, length of stay, and itinerary. However, some basic items we like to include are a camera, film (and extra batteries), a small rubber door wedge to place under the hotel guestroom door, small flashlight for emergencies, and a plastic clothes bag for dirty socks and underwear unless your suitcase has an extra compartment. Don't forget to take a battery-operated smoke detector if traveling to areas where they are not provided in your room. We also like to take a small sewing kit that includes a couple of safety pins.

Packing to Return Home

Items that can be easily replaced at home, such as toiletries and first aid kit, can be placed in your checked baggage for your return flights. If you are traveling internationally and have purchased souvenirs, place these together in your carry-on bag if they are lightweight or valuable. When traveling internationally, you will need to keep track of all items purchased while outside the U.S. and prepare a list for returning through U.S. Customs. Don't forget to pack an envelope to keep receipts separate. Packing all items together in one bag will make the process easier should Customs agents request to see any of your purchases. Place your envelope with a list of all purchases in the bags with the items. You will need to list the item and the cost of each item in U.S. dollars.

8

Your Personal Safety Guide

Personal safety *should* become a lifestyle. Learning and practicing good safety habits on a daily basis will help enable you to protect yourself without living in fear. Habits such as carrying your purse properly and always locking doors should become second nature to you. The more confident you are in your safety and well being, the more you will enjoy your travel experience.

So how do you make "personal safety a lifestyle"? The key to practicing good safety habits without fear is to think of yourself as a confident traveling woman, not a potential target. This will help project an image that you are self-assured and may actually draw less attention from someone who may be searching for a victim. For example, a pickpocket will want to get to your wallet in as little time as possible and move on. So the key is to make it difficult and "too much trouble" for them to bother with you.

Sergeant Michael Janin, a personal-defense training expert for the City of Beaverton police department in Oregon, advises women to use "tactical awareness." Sergeant Janin explains, "Tactical awareness is knowing that you have a rehearsed plan that you know you can act on if needed. Just as we learn CPR in case of emergency, women need to know how to protect themselves before getting into a situation where their personal safety is threatened."

Janin, who has over 20 years experience in coaching women on personal-defense tactics, shares some basic tips for women travelers:

- *Always* stay aware of your surroundings; your mind should be on what you are doing, not on what you 'll say to Aunt Martha when you get off the plane.

- Make eye contact with people when traveling; criminals do not want you to be able to identify them.

- Criminals will look for an easy target; make it difficult for them so they will move on.

- Keep your hands free; women are more vulnerable when their hands are bound up in straps of purses and bags.

- Don't place yourself in a vulnerable situation; stand and sit in areas where you will have an escape route should you need it such as airport waiting areas and restaurants.

- Know that the universal gesture for "STOP" is a palm up facing the person; use this if someone is getting too close to you.

- Be verbal; talk loudly if you feel threatened, as this will control your breathing and release energy to help you gain control of the situation.

- If you are followed in a parking lot, bang on cars to set off alarms.

- When getting in an elevator, stand next to the controls facing the door.

- If you are uncomfortable in an elevator, hit the buttons on all floors an get out as soon as possible; state loudly that you are looking for your husband who was lifting weights in the gym.

Sergeant Janin's advice to women is to contact their local police department to ask about personal defense workshops offered in their area. "Many women think of self-defense as learning karate or fighting tactics," Janin says. "Personal defense is understanding tactical awareness and ways to prevent placing yourself in a vulnerable situation. You will have more confidence traveling if you develop a rehearsed plan on how you would deal with a situation if confronted."

As you learn that protecting yourself does not mean clutching your purse as you dart through throngs of pedestrians like a football player attacking opponents, but, rather, carrying yourself with an air of confidence, you will become more comfortable traveling. Walking with your hand draped comfortably on a purse slung across your torso can keep your hands free and protect your belongings without paranoia. Once you learn how to do this without thinking about it, you can actually relax and become more aware of what is going on around you. The goal is to be comfortable in your surroundings as you travel, whether walking down a busy New York street or touring the Louvre in Paris.

Being Comfortable in a Strange Place

The more comfortable you can become while traveling, the more you will reduce the fear of being in a strange place.

Consul General Larry Colbert of the U.S. Consulate in Paris, France, encourages travelers to be aware of their surroundings at all times. "It is common for travelers in a foreign country to be taken with the quaintness of the area and let their barriers down," he says. "They may think, 'nothing can happen to me here'." He suggests traveling lightly and leaving valuables at home. "I recommend using hotel safes to store airline tickets, passports, and extra credit cards. Carry only one credit card and a small amount of cash when you are out for the day."

Mr. Colbert has served in consulates in seven countries and regularly deals with travelers who have had valuables stolen. "They come into the Consulate on a daily basis, distraught over losing their wallet, passport, purse, etc. It is common to have U.S. citizens come to our office within 24 hours of arriving in France. Most of these thefts happen on public transportation when travelers first arrive and are so busy with finding transportation and being in a foreign country that they are not paying attention to their belongings." He advises, "Consider taking a taxi from the airport rather than public transportation, particularly if traveling with a great deal of luggage. A traveler is tired after a long international flight, often disoriented in a foreign country, and has to keep track of bags, carry-ons, passport, and money, etc., making the individual all too vulnerable to thieves." Mr. Colbert's top travel tips are:

- Take a taxi from the airport instead of public transportation because it is safer when transporting luggage.

- Never lock valuables in the trunk of a rental car, as thieves can easily break into trunks.

- When dining out late at night, ask the restaurant staff to call a taxi to take you back to your hotel.

- Make sure hotel room doors have deadbolts.

- Keep valuables in the hotel safe and only take what you need for the day.

Protecting Yourself While Traveling

Beware of Pickpockets

Whether just starting your journey at your hometown airport, or in the middle of a tour in a foreign country, pickpockets can be a threat. Tour coordinator Jim Boehner encourages his clients to wear a hidden money belt and never put valuables in backpacks or fanny-packs, "They are just too vulnerable in crowds," Jim states. "I also suggest that they keep an extra credit card and cash in a separate place such as an inside zipper pocket." He speaks from personal experience. While escorting a tour in Venice, Jim was standing at an ice cream stand when a woman approached him. "She was carrying a baby in one arm and as she leaned toward me, I suddenly felt a hand reach for my pocket! I realized that she had a wooden arm holding the baby and an opening in her coat in which she could slide her hand out to pick a pocket." Jim's advice: "Always be protective of your valuables and be aware of your surroundings." He cautions travelers to be especially careful if there is a distraction. "Anytime there is a distraction, watch out for pickpockets." Thieves will use various methods to get your attention while a co-conspirator will grab your valuables. One of Jim's clients was pickpocketed at the Metro in Paris when a group of kids created a distraction by jumping the turnstile, while another kid relieved him of his wallet.

Women especially can be vulnerable to pickpockets and purse-snatchers because thieves may use distractions that play on our emotions. Expert thieves will create diversions using children that will cause a woman traveler to forget about protecting her valuables long enough for the thief to steal them. They may do things like throw a baby in your arms to distract you or use children to surround you begging and clinging so close that you may not feel someone reaching into your purse.

Pickpockets often work in pairs or groups and are experts at targeting victims, distracting them and stealing their purse or wallet. They are usually after money, but because many travelers carry their cash, credit cards, and identification such as passports in one place, the thief gets it all. We recommend that you always carry your valuables in various places, such as a money belt and an inside zippered pocket, with only those necessary items needed for the day in your purse.

Patricia Mounier, corporate communication officer at the Louvre in Paris, encourages women to carry small handbags with the opening facing their body. They post warnings to help visitors become aware of potential pickpockets and even have plainclothes security agents on duty. However, there is still a risk if travelers are not paying attention to their belongings. "Visitors will be preoccupied with viewing the art or taking pictures and forget to protect their purse," she says.

Traveling by Air

Air travel has increased dramatically in the last ten years, and indications are that more and more people will choose to travel by air in the future. While traveling by plane, most of us tend to think of safety only in terms of the airplane itself and whether we will land without any problems. There are, however, precautions that you should take to protect your belongings while traveling on a plane, especially on long flights when you want to get up and walk around, visit the restroom, or sleep. We interviewed women who arrived at their destination only to realize that their wallet had been stolen from their purse sometime during their flight. It is easy to protect your bags while flying if you practice the same safety habits you would while in any public venue. We choose to wear our money belts while traveling, even on a plane, because they are comfortable and your valuables are protected at all times. If you need to get up to use the restroom, take your purse with you. If you are traveling with a companion, ask him/her to keep an eye on it for you.

Safety at the Airport

Airport layovers, flight delays, and cancellations are realities in today's travel world. Staying safe and comfortable while waiting for flights is easier today with the amenities offered at many major airports. Keep an eye on your carry-on while waiting in airports. Unattended bags are vulnerable to thieves.

Monique Bond, an assistant commissioner of media relations for a major U.S. airport, encourages travelers to protect their bags at all times. "Think of the airport as a city within a city," Monique says. "If you remove the roof from the airport facility, the environment is as open and vulnerable as a downtown city. Most women would not stand on a street corner in a busy downtown area and set their bags and purses on the ground next to them while looking at maps, etc., but we see that all the time in airports. People have a tendency to think that, because they are in an enclosed building, they are safer, but airports are public places and travelers need to be careful with their belongings."

When going through airport security, keep an eye on your bags when placing them on the x-ray belt. Make sure that you can get to your bag quickly after passing through the metal detector. While traveling internationally, make sure that outside pockets on bags are zipped. Not only are bags vulnerable for thieves to rob, but can also be a target for smugglers who may place drugs or other illegal items in the bag of a fellow passenger and then steal it when they arrive at the destination. The police and Customs officials have a right to search your luggage for drugs or other suspected illegal items. If they find these in your suitcase, you will suffer the consequences. While dining, waiting at the gate, or using the restroom, do not leave your bag unattended. If you feel that your bag has been out of your control while waiting at the airport, report it immediately to airport security. Also, do not agree to carry a package for anyone, no matter how small it might seem.

During long layovers, you may be tempted to leave the airport in search of sightseeing, shopping, or culinary opportunities. The safest place for you will most likely be at the airport. Many of today's airports offer a variety of shops and restaurants to wile away the hours. If you are determined to leave, use common sense. Ask yourself these questions: Are you familiar with the area? Do you speak the language? Is there safe transportation available? Are you assured of returning in time to catch your plane? Your most important consideration is your safety!

Safety at Your Hotel

When checking in, register under your last name and first initial. Ask the agent to give you your room number discreetly so that others cannot overhear. If you are traveling alone, ask for an escort to your room such as the bellman. It is a good idea to let the bellman handle your bags rather trying to manage luggage on your own. It is safer for you not to be dragging luggage down the hotel corridors, not to mention easier on your arms and back.

Do not be afraid to ask about the safety of your room. Ask if the room has a deadbolt lock. Keep your key secured and out of sight at all times. Many hotels in foreign countries will keep your hotel key at the front desk in a box with the room number labeled on it in plain view. When asking for your key, take care who may overhear you stating your room number. Again, if you are uncomfortable for any reason, ask for someone to walk you to your room and wait until you are safely inside. Do not be afraid to refuse a room if you are not comfortable with your safety.

When getting settled into your room, check the locks on windows and doors to make sure they work properly. Orient yourself with fire safety procedures such as where the emergency exits are located and escape routes. Check to make sure that the smoke detector is working. Some seasoned travelers suggest counting the number of doors from your room to the emergency stairwell. This could be critical if you need to find your way through a smoke-filled corridor.

While in your room, keep the deadbolt locked at all times. We recommend carrying a small door wedge and keeping it tucked under the door, or using an alarm that can be set to go off if someone opens the door. You can find these at travel and luggage stores. Never open the door to a stranger. Rooms with a one-way viewer are the safest for identifying someone at the door. If you order room service, confirm that the person is hotel staff before opening the door. If you are uncertain that they are hotel staff, call the front desk for verification. Do not hang the "Make up Room" sign on the door handle; this will draw attention to the fact that you are not in your room. Instead, call the front desk to request housekeeping services. Also avoid using the door sign provided to order food service. This would allow anyone reading the sign to know that you are ordering for one person only. Call the room service number to order meals instead. When you leave for the evening, hang the "Do Not Disturb" sign on your door so that anyone passing by will think you are in your room.

Dressing for the Day

We have discussed recommended clothing in Chapter Seven, "Packing With Safety and Health in Mind." However, when choosing your daily wardrobe, dress appropriately for the places you will be visiting that day. While you may have packed your best little print dress for an evening out, it would not be appropriate for a day touring cathedrals or attending a business meeting. Many foreign countries have strict protocol in how women should dress and present themselves. While interviewing travel professionals in France, we were told that American women stand out because typically Americans are very open and friendly and dress more casually than their French peers. This, they said, can make a woman stand out as a tourist and a target for pickpockets. Review your itinerary for the day and dress accordingly. Dressing conservatively while traveling can help you look less like a tourist. Try to fit in with the locals and not stand out by your attire.

In some countries, behavior that we would consider as sexual harassment in the U.S. may be common, especially on public transportation. Men may stare at you or make suggestive statements. If you find yourself in this situation, ignore the verbal comments unless you are physically touched, in which case you should yell loudly. When in public, stand or sit near other women and try not to draw attention to yourself.

Jewelry

We have already discussed the wisdom of traveling with little jewelry, but, you may have packed jewelry for special occasions or purchased new jewelry to take home. While not wearing it, keep your items in the hotel safe. Many hotels now provide safes in the room. You can usually set your own combination to the lock and have access to it as many times as you wish. When placing items in the hotel office safe, remember to ask for a receipt listing what items you left there. If going to a party, keep your jewelry out of sight until you arrive at your destination, especially if taking public transportation. For example, if you are wearing a coat, button it up until you reach the party.

Walking Around

If possible, always walk in pairs. Use routes that will lead you through well-trafficked areas and public places. Avoid walking close to buildings that have alcoves where someone may be standing, hidden from view, especially at night. Avoid consulting a map while standing on a street. Instead, plan your route before you leave your hotel. Walk with confidence and purpose, and avoid eye contact with strangers. If you need to walk alone, try to avoid looking like a tourist or visitor, as these are prime targets for pickpockets and purse-snatchers. If you get lost, need directions, or need to consult your map, step into a building. Ask for directions from store clerks or police officers rather than from a stranger. Be cautious when crossing streets and do not assume that in foreign countries a pedestrian has the right-of-way, as is the case in most American states.

Dining Out

When dining in a restaurant, keep your purse next to you where you can see it. Avoid hanging it on the back of your chair. Take care when giving your credit card to the restaurant staff that you receive your own card back. If dining late at night, ask the restaurant staff to call a taxi for you.

Dealing with Beggars

It has become a common sight in cities around the world to see beggars asking for money. This is especially prevalent in tourist areas of many foreign countries. Beggars use many tactics to induce your sympathy. They will sit along the side of the road with children and ask for help to feed their babies, or they will walk up to visitors and ask for change. Many beggars also use children to do the asking, and it is common in some countries to be followed by a group of children asking for money. They will target women because women tend to be more emotional by nature and, therefore, more sympathetic. Our advice is don't give them anything! We have talked to travelers who carry candy or pencils, etc. in their pocket and hand this to the children;

however, you then risk being hounded by groups of children as you try to walk down the street. There are many charities and churches that assist the poor, and we recommend giving your donations through a reputable organization.

Also, be aware of street vendors. Not only will opening your purse on the street make you more vulnerable to purse snatchers or pickpockets, but many of the items for sale are actually scams. Products from street vendors are seldom the quality the vendor is advertising. Upon arrival in a new area, check with hotel staff or local authorities to inquire as to whether street vendors are authorized merchants.

Carrying Your Currency and Making Transactions

We have talked about carrying your credit cards, extra money, passport, etc. in a hidden money belt, but, when you are going on a tour, sightseeing, shopping, or on your way to a meeting, you will need some cash or a credit card handy. We suggest that you carry enough cash or a credit card, phone card, etc. that you will need for the day and place it in a small purse that you can wear diagonally across your torso. This will allow you to have your money at hand and protect it at the same time. There are a variety of bags available with long straps, and most are lightweight yet roomy enough to also carry other small necessities you may need for the day.

Representatives of the American Consulate in Paris warn that many U.S. citizens become a target for theft while at currency exchange bureaus. They have seen time and again people who will walk up and down the street looking at all the exchange rates searching for the lowest rate. They will sometimes see people going back and forth when the difference may only be a few percentage points. What many travelers do not realize is that professional thieves know how to identify tourists and may be watching. Once they target you as a tourist, they will search for ways to separate you from your cash. Many women also become careless with their purse while making a transaction. They may have a tendency to leave their purse gaping open or set aside while exchanging currency. Thieves have many tricks they use. In some foreign countries, women will use tricks such as throwing a doll, wrapped to look like a baby, at a woman tourist who has her purse open while making a purchase. Usually the shocked tourist will grab for the "baby" and leave her purse vulnerable for the thief to seize and run. Our advice is to be aware of your surroundings at all times and keep your belongings close to you during any transaction. Be discreet and never flash large amounts of cash while traveling.

When making a transaction, be aware of where your credit card is at all times. Make sure the card returned to you is *your* card. After a purchase, replace your credit card back in its secure location along with the receipt. The receipt is critical because it may list your credit card number on it and you will also need it for Customs upon re-entry to the U.S. Take your time when making credit card transactions, as many crimes occur when the victim is in a hurry. Becoming flustered may cause carelessness and could place you in a vulnerable situation. If you find that your credit card has been lost or stolen, immediately contact your provider.

Carrying Your Passport

Many travel experts suggest carrying a copy of your passport with you in your money belt and leaving your original passport in your hotel safe, but it is becoming increasingly common for merchants, banks, etc. to require passport identification to make a transaction. Some merchants will ask for your passport as identification when you make a purchase using a credit card or travelers checks. Foreign currency exchange bureaus and banks will most likely ask you for your passport when making a transaction, especially those involving use of a credit card. If you will need your passport, carry it with you, and leave the photocopy in the hotel safe. Most pickpockets are looking for money and are not interested in passports, although there is still a large black market for passports throughout the world. If your passport is lost or stolen, immediately report it to the police and ask for a copy of the police report. Take the report to the nearest U.S. Consulate office for assistance in replacing your passport or obtaining necessary travel documents. (How to access the Consulate is explained in Chapter Nine, "Dealing with Problems and Emergencies.")

Conversing with Travel Companions and Strangers

Knowing the protocol of your destination area will help you to become more comfortable in conversation. For example, in France, a customer is expected to greet shop owners when entering. This can be fun, especially if you learn a few words such as *bonjour*. Shop owners and local residents can be a great source of information. They will most likely know the best places to eat, the not-to-miss sites, and easiest way to get around. Walk into a nearby shop to ask for directions instead of asking someone on the street. As mentioned before, avoid studying a map in public; instead seek help in a place of business or from a police officer.

When talking with travel companions, be aware of your surroundings and who may be overhearing your conversation. Take care not to reveal personal information out loud, especially where you are staying and your itinerary. Never give out personal information to strangers. This can happen innocently when talking with people at airports, restaurants, etc., and you become engaged in a conversation in which someone may ask, "Oh, where are you staying? I know the area well." Before you know it, you can give out information that may make you vulnerable to criminals. It is better to answer by saying the general area in which you are staying instead of naming the hotel.

Don't accept invitations from strangers who may offer you a ride or ask you to a party. If you are looking for places to enjoy the local nightlife, ask the concierge at the hotel to recommend a place and take a taxi there and back.

Using Public Transportation and Taxis

Once you arrive at your destination, you will need local transportation to get around. Again, it is advisable to know ahead of time how to find reputable service providers. Your hotel representative may be able to direct you to public transportation.

Subways: In many large cities, subways are the most common form of public transportation. Unfortunately, subways can also be insecure places for personal safety. A young woman who was molested while on a subway in Mexico learned how vulnerable one can be in such a situation. She was on a crowded train and did not even see her attacker. If possible, avoid traveling at peak times when trains are packed. This can be tricky, however, because usually the peak times are when daily workers are commuting and can be a safer environment, so try to travel when you know that there will be other regular commuters. Avoid traveling on subways late at night; a taxi may be a safer choice. When boarding a subway, keep your belongings in front of you with a firm grip. Do not wear a backpack on your back while in a subway or crowded area, as these have been a target for thieves who have cut the bottom out without the victim being aware. Take your backpack off and hold it securely in front of you. If you must stand, stay close to the door or wall. If you are violated in any way, yell loudly and draw attention. Go to the nearest police or security office as soon as possible.

Buses: When getting on a bus, sit toward the front near the driver. Keep purse and bags firmly placed in your lap with openings facing toward you. Be aware of who may be watching as you get off the bus, and if for any reason you do not feel comfortable, wait on the bus until the next stop. Look for stops that are well lit and take the time while riding to get your keys ready if you are going to a parked car. Knowing the route ahead of time will help you know what to expect when traveling around a city by bus. If you are traveling on a tour bus, keep your valuables with you at all times. When the bus stops at designated rest areas, do not leave your belongings on the bus unless you are confident that the driver will lock the bus while the tour group is using the facilities or eating, etc.

Taxis: Do not assume that taxi drivers will know the way back to your hotel, especially if they do not speak your language. One good suggestion is to go to the front desk of your hotel upon check-in and get a card with the name and directions to the hotel in the language of the country you are visiting. You can then show this to the driver (make sure he doesn't keep it). However, it is still advisable to know the route so that you can make sure you are going in the right direction.

If, at any time, you are uncomfortable with the driving method or the direction in which you are going, tell the driver to either please slow down or request to be dropped off.

While escorting a delegation to South Korea, Catherine and a travel companion, Nina, were taking a taxi from downtown Seoul to the airport. They later describe the ride as "...one of the most terrifying taxi rides we have ever taken! The driver sped through the streets, narrowly missing oncoming cars and almost hitting a bus. We were really shaken by the time we arrived at the airport."

If faced with this situation, ask the driver to let you out as soon as you feel you are in a safe location to be dropped off, such as a busy street corner where you can find another taxi. Trust your instincts! Your safety is the most important issue.

When arriving at a destination with luggage, be aware if the driver opens the trunk before you get out of the car. Thieves have been known to grab luggage out of the trunk of a taxi before the driver or passenger gets out of the car.

Trains: We have mentioned the popularity of traveling by train in many foreign countries.

Three female students whom we interviewed in France were traveling around Europe by train. Dawn, Natalie, and Kristen were young students from Wisconsin who experienced many delights of traveling by train and seeing the European country-side, but they also had some experiences in which they were not comfortable with their safety. Boarding trains in which they were the only female passengers happened more than once. They adopted the policy of always staying close together when they traveled. They were careful not to be too friendly with strangers and kept a close eye on their luggage at all times.

Traveling with a group is the safest method of any kind of travel, but if you find that you need to travel alone or with another female, try to book your trip during the day when trains are busy with other tourists or business travelers. Keep your belongings close to you at all times and report any problems or concerns to the conductor.

Using Rental Cars

When picking up a rental car, examine the exterior and interior and point out any dents, scratches, etc. to the agent. Do not accept a rental car without noting these items on the rental agreement. When you first get into a rental car, orient yourself to the devices. Find the headlight switch, window buttons, wipers, etc., so that you will avoid driving down the freeway frantically looking for the windshield wipers during a sudden rainstorm. While inside a rental car, always keep your doors locked. Keep maps and car rental agreements out of site, especially when leaving the car. Do not leave any items visible that may target you as a tourist and do not lock valuables in a rental car, not

 even in the trunk. In many foreign countries, rental car agencies register all rental cars under a certain code using a beginning set of numbers that are consistent. Many organized thieves know these codes and can target a car as a rental. Cars can be broken into in a matter of seconds so always check the interior before getting in.

Driving

First of all, *always* buckle your seat belt. If someone in a car next to you tells you that something is wrong with your vehicle or is flashing their headlights, do not stop. Go to the nearest service station or stop at a well-populated area. Use the same advice if someone bumps you from behind. If you have a cell phone, call the police as soon as you feel you can. Many carjackings happen while sitting at stoplights; therefore, do not drive right up to the back of the vehicle in front of you. Leave plenty of room in case you must pull away quickly. Always keep doors locked and windows rolled up when driving in congested places.

As lonely as you may become out on that highway with many miles ahead, do not succumb to the idea of picking up a hitchhiker, as this is very dangerous, especially if traveling alone. Be mindful of pedestrians, as they will walk out in front of you even when it is not their turn. In some foreign countries you could face stiff penalties and sometimes jail time for hitting a pedestrian.

Never park near vans, as this is an easy way to become a victim. If you find that someone has parked near your car, you may want to enter your car from the passenger side. When you approach your vehicle, just take a quick peak underneath to make sure no one is hiding.

When you are in your car using the ATM, make sure you are in a very well-lit area and that there are no bushes or obstructions that may hide someone who could rob you. Roll your window up before counting your money.

If you have a breakdown, *do not* accept assistance from anyone. In Seattle a few years ago, there was an incident during rush hour traffic, when a woman had car problems and pulled to the side of the road. A man pulled over to see if there was a problem and she made herself vulnerable to him by getting out of her car. He proceeded to make her get into the back of the car and raped her. You should have an emergency kit in your car and a sign that says "Call Police." If someone approaches your vehicle, tell them to phone the police. You can do this without rolling down your window.

Never stop your car to help someone on the side of the road. Pull into the nearest exit and call the police and report the disabled vehicle.

Using a Public Restroom

Always try to choose a restroom in a public building or facility. If possible, try to avoid going down deserted hallways. Always lock the door. When you are in the restroom, do not hang your purse over the hook provided on the back of the door unless it is secured. If you must set your purse or bag on the floor, set it directly in front of your feet where it cannot be reached from outside the stall. If traveling in foreign countries, keep in mind that public restroom facilities are not necessarily the same as in the United States. In many countries, you will have to pay an attendant or insert coins before entering, so remember to carry change with you as you leave for the day. Always carry a small pack of tissue, as it is very common to find restrooms out of toilet paper. Another good tip is to carry a small packet of antibacterial wipes for disinfecting your hands as not all toilets provide hot water and soap. It is common in some large cities, to have public restrooms right on the sidewalk. You insert a coin to enter, and when you leave there can be a disinfectant spray that comes down from the ceiling, so take care not to hold the door open for someone else to enter. You must deposit a coin for each person using the facility.

Keeping in Touch with Home

U.S. State Department representatives recommend checking in with home contacts periodically, especially if traveling for longer than two weeks or if you are going to vary from your itinerary.

Safety on a Cruise

As with airlines, the cruise ships have a safety instruction announcement that you should pay careful attention to. It will tell you where and how to get to the lifeboats and where the life vests are and how to fasten them. A whistle and light are attached to the vest, and you need to know how to access them in case of emergency. Don't assume that because you are on a contained vessel you do not need to lock your cabin doors. Treat your cabin as you would a hotel room: keep your stateroom door locked and identify a visitor before opening it.

Follow the safety tips for walking around and using transportation while visiting ports. Also take care to protect your valuables when ashore as these tourist destinations are prepared for the cruise ship passengers and can be a venue for pickpockets, purse snatchers, beggars, and scam artists. They know that cruise passengers will be coming into the port to shop and will most likely be carrying cash and credit cards.

9

Dealing with Problems and Emergencies

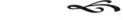

What to Do if Faced With a Crisis

Even with careful planning, incidents can occur while traveling—problems ranging from small nuisances and discomforts to actual emergencies. Whom would you call if you became ill on a trip? What do you do if you are the victim of a crime? Where would you go if you lost your passport?

Knowing ahead of time how to find help when problems or emergencies occur can save precious time and frustration if actually faced with an incident. If traveling on business, obtain phone numbers of business contacts at their office or home whom you can call in case an emergency occurs.

Traveler's Woes

Your luggage is lost: Immediately report lost luggage to the airline. Chances are good that your luggage will be located and the airline will deliver it to you. It will help if you can give the airline an accurate description of your bag other than a black roll-on-board, which is what just about every person traveling seems to use nowadays. If you have placed a colorful ribbon or tag on your bag, be sure to describe it. Hopefully you have placed an identification tag on the outside of your bag and a copy on the inside. Know what your rights are in requesting that they provide temporary items such as toiletries and clothing, especially if you have an important meeting, etc., and need items immediately.

> *When faced with an emergency, try to remain calm and take one step at a time*

You have lost your airline tickets: Immediately call the local office of the airline company and report the loss. Whenever possible it is advisable to use electronic tickets to avoid the danger of having paper tickets lost or stolen, but this is not always possible. Ask the airline if they can replace your ticket. If possible, go to the airport or airline office immediately and present identification.

You suffer traveler's illnesses: If you become ill or are injured but do not require emergency attention, try to get back to where you are staying. Ask your host or hotel staff for assistance.

Emergencies

Emergency aid professionals tell us that the first thing to do when an emergency occurs is try not to panic. Remain calm and take one step at a time. Look for the nearest source of help.

Life-Threatening Emergencies

Domestic travel: While traveling domestically, you will be able to find emergency assistance quickly because of the U.S. emergency response system. We know to call 911 inside the U.S. for police, fire, and medical assistance.

International travel: Emergencies while traveling internationally bring a whole new set of concerns because there is no standard number to call. Each country has its own contact numbers and process for dealing with emergencies. Ask local residents, hotel staff, etc. for numbers to call.

You are injured or become ill: Seek medical attention immediately; however, unless you are too ill to make a decision, wait until you completely understand what procedures you are agreeing to. If traveling internationally, ask the medical staff to call the U.S. Consulate. They will be able to provide assistance such as an interpreter to translate discussions with your doctor if necessary, contact your doctor at home, and call friends or family for you.

You have been the victim of a crime: Most authorities tell us not to fight if we are mugged, because attackers very often carry knives and we can become injured. They do tell us though that we should make as much noise as possible. Scream loudly (usually yelling "Fire" is recommended). Immediately call the local police and file a report. The important issue is your safety, so make sure you are safe first before worrying about your belongings. If a crime occurs in your hotel, ask the hotel management to call the police for you. Try to remain calm and give authorities as many details as possible to assist them in catching the person or persons. Ask to be moved to another room. Call a family member or friend at home. It can be very comforting to hear a familiar voice in times of crisis.

Non Life-Threatening Emergencies

You have an emergency at home and need to return: Most airline companies will be as helpful as possible when travelers are facing emergency situations. They will try to accommodate your request to change airline reservations; however, keep in mind that some companies have strict policies regarding charges for changing a reservation. The safest precaution is to take out travelers insurance before you go, especially if you have a loved one at home who is ill and may face an emergency requiring you to return home quickly.

Your money or credit cards have been lost or stolen: Report your loss to the local police and obtain a copy of your report. Immediately contact the credit card company. If traveling domestically, call the toll-free number and report your loss. When traveling internationally, some consulates can provide local access numbers of major credit card companies. If you cannot find one, ask for directory assistance for the U.S. Most major companies will have 24-hour phone assistance for lost or stolen cards. Ask for a replacement card. If all of your money has been stolen and you have no way to get money from an ATM machine, or don't have another credit card, you can have money wired to you through a number of agencies. Ask local authorities which companies can assist you.

Finding Help

Domestic Assistance

Organizations such as Travelers Aid International can provide assistance to travelers in need of help through information and referral booths in airports or bus stations. The center that we visited was located in Chicago O'Hare Airport where the staff offered everything from a band-aid, to directions, to assisting elderly travelers. According to Ray Flynt, President of Travelers Aid International, there are Travelers Aid agencies or programs in about 55 communities across the U.S. The list of programs can be found on their website, *www.travelersaid.org*. Travelers Aid centers are located in 23 airports around the country and at a few additional transportation centers such as train and bus stations.

Mr. Flynt adds, "Travelers Aid's historic mission is to help stranded and disconnected people. In that sense, we do our best to reconnect people with their own resources (helping them with a phone call, to arrange for transfer of funds, etc.). For persons in dire straits, Travelers Aid can possibly provide transportation assistance to help get them home. All decisions regarding assistance offered are made at the local level. At airport locations, much of the assistance provided is in the form of information. For example, telling people about the various alternatives for ground transportation to get from an airport into a city. Generally there are no fees for service. In some of the airport locations Travelers Aid provides assistance to meet elderly persons and help get them from one airline to another. They may charge for this service since it needs to be arranged in advance."

Contacts When Traveling Internationally

If an emergency occurs while traveling abroad, the American Services Office of the Consulate at the U.S. Embassy can be your best resource. There are U.S. embassies in more than 160 capital cities of the world. Each embassy has a consular section. There are also consular officers at about 60 U.S. consulates general and 20 U.S. consulates around the world. (Consulates general and consulates are regional offices of embassies.) Local employees who are citizens of the host country usually assist U.S. consuls. These locals are valuable in helping with translations and contacts. We encourage you to visit the consulate, if you have the time, when you travel to a foreign country. This will familiarize you with their location as well as with what they offer U.S. citizens living or traveling abroad.

Getting Help at the Consulate

The American Services Office (ASO) of the consulate is staffed with sympathetic personnel who realize that you have, most likely, just gone through a trying situation since you are walking through their doors. They will be as accommodating as possible and can offer a variety of solution options.

When you arrive at the consulate, you will be asked to walk through a security checkpoint. Be prepared to have your U.S. passport ready if you have it. Since the number one problem U.S. citizens bring to the consulate while traveling is theft of passports, they will understand if you are there because your passport was lost or stolen. Bring any identification that you do have. If you have none, you may bring a friend or relative with you who has his/her own identification and can vouch for your identity.

As you enter the consulate offices, you will be greeted by a receptionist, who will ask you the nature of your business. You will then be directed to the area and personnel who can help you.

While researching this book, we were invited to the American Consulate in Paris to meet with staff of the American Services Office. They invited us to come to the office on a Monday morning to observe the regular group of American citizens who had been robbed over the weekend. As these travelers came in for help, they almost always had the same story: they were robbed of their, purse, wallet, etc. while on public transportation or walking around the city. Most of them told us that they just did not think about getting robbed and did not take proper precautions in protecting their valuables. Women who had their wallet, passport, etc. taken out of their purse without their knowing it was a common practice.

We spoke with a young woman who was residing in Florence for a year on an exchange program through school. She was on a two-week break and had come to Paris on a train with some friends. They had to change trains in Pisa, Italy, and boarded the Paris-bound train at 2:45am. She said the train was crowded and there was a lot of confusion during the transfer when, all of a sudden, she felt her belongings falling out of her backpack. She believes that as she bent over to retrieve the items her wallet was stolen. Her passport as well as her cash was in the wallet. She reported the theft to police and came to the consulate to have her passport replaced.

We asked her if she considered wearing a money belt. She told us. "My mother and I had that very conversation before I left Florence." She said that since she was living in Europe, traveled quite a bit, and was not going very far, she really let her guard down. When asked how she would travel differently since her experience, she said, "I will be purchasing and wearing a money belt."

What the Consulate Can Do:

Replace a passport: If you lose your passport, a consul can issue you a replacement, often within 24 hours. If you believe your passport has been stolen, first report the theft to the local police and get a police declaration.

Help find medical assistance: If you get sick, you can contact a consular officer for a list of local doctors, dentists, and medical specialists, along with other medical information. If you are injured or become seriously ill, a consul will help you find medical assistance and, at your request, inform your family or friends. (Consider getting private medical insurance before you travel, to cover the high cost of getting you back to the U.S. for hospital care in the event of a medical emergency.)

Help get funds: Should you lose all your money and other financial resources, consular officers can help you contact your family, bank, or employer to arrange for them to send you funds. In some cases, these funds can be wired to you through the State Department.

Help in an emergency: Your family may need to reach you because of an emergency at home or because they are worried about your welfare. They should call the State Department's Overseas Citizens Services at 202-647-5225. The State Department will relay the message to the consular officers in the country in which you are traveling. Consular officers will attempt to locate you, pass on urgent messages, and, consistent with the Privacy Act, report back to your family.

Visit in jail: If you are arrested, you should ask the authorities to notify a U.S. consul. Consuls cannot get you out of jail (when you are in a foreign country you are subject to its laws). However, they can work to protect your legitimate interests and ensure you are not discriminated against. They can provide a list of local attorneys, visit you, inform you generally about local laws, and contact your family and friends. Consular officers can transfer money, food, and clothing to the prison authorities from your family or friends. They can try to get relief if you are held under inhumane or unhealthful conditions.

Make arrangements after the death of an American: When an American dies abroad, a consular officer notifies the American's family and informs them about options and costs for disposition of remains. Costs for preparing and returning a body to the U.S. may be high and must be paid by the family. Often, local laws and procedures make returning a body to the U.S. for burial a lengthy process. A consul prepares a Report of Death based on the local death certificate; this is forwarded to the next of kin for use in estate and insurance matters.

Help in a disaster/evacuation: If you are caught up in a natural disaster or civil disturbance, you should let your relatives know as soon as possible that you are safe, or contact a U.S. consul who will pass that message to your family through the State Department. Be resourceful. U.S. officials will do everything they can to contact you and advise you. However, they must give priority to helping Americans who have been hurt or are in immediate danger. In a disaster, consuls face the same constraints you do; lack of electricity or fuel, interrupted phone lines, and closed airports.

What Consular Officers Cannot Do

In addition to the qualifications noted above, consular officers cannot act as travel agents, bankers, lawyers, investigators, or law enforcement officers. Please do not expect them to find you employment, get you residence or driving permits, act as interpreters, search for missing luggage, or settle disputes with hotel managers. They can, however, tell you how to get help on these and other matters.

Most of us will never deal with major emergencies while traveling; however, when an emergency occurs, it can be critical to be prepared. Before you go, find out as much information as possible such as insurance company phone numbers and names of emergency service providers at your destination. Sometimes just knowing where the local police station or consulate is located can be your best source during an emergency.

10

Our Favorite Websites for Women Travelers

Travel planning on the Internet has never been easier with thousands of websites available. We have identified some of our favorite sites for helping women travelers. Many of the sites are designed for women by women. Other sites are great resources for finding basic information such as what to expect when traveling internationally or road conditions when taking a cross-country excursion. For the business traveler, find out protocol for doing business in foreign countries. We have also listed sites that let you network with women around the world. Many sites have links that will lead you to additional resources. Enjoy browsing and remember to keep your health and safety in mind as you plan your trip!

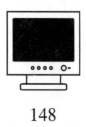

Especially for Women Travelers

Her Mail
www.hermail.net

This is one of our favorite sites for networking with women around the world. You register and submit your email address and their database will provide you with two email addresses of women that have registered with HerMail in the location you are researching. It has tips and articles for and about women.

Journeywoman™
www.journeywoman.com

Journeywoman.com is designed for women travelers and includes a free newsletter and articles featuring women's adventures around the world. The site is user friendly, a great resource for the woman who travels or is thinking about travel, and covers international issues as well as domestic concerns.

Women Business Travelers
www.womenbusinesstravelers.com

This site, operated by Wyndham Hotels and Resorts, is focused on the woman business traveler and the concerns she might encounter while traveling. It provides ideas on dressing for travel comfort that tips that will make her trip easier and more enjoyable.

Women's Travel Club
www.womenstravelclub.com

This is a site "Designed for Women by Women" and is a membership site; for a nominal fee per year you can access its tours.

It does, however, have some great articles and offers advice on travel that is available to all.

Women.com
www.women.com/travel/

This is a site that all women will enjoy. There is something for everyone. The travel page contains articles as well as the latest hot spots and what to do while there. The site merged with iVillage.com, but has retained its name.

Senior Women
www.seniorwomen.com/travel.htm

Great site for seniors wanting to find out where and how to travel with ease. There are great articles for frequent travelers as well as those who have some difficulty traveling or getting around. You can also submit your travel experiences or opinions.

Websites for Researching Your Destination

U.S. State Department
www.state.gov

This is our favorite reference site for U.S. citizens who plan on traveling abroad. In addition to up-to-date information about travel advisories for countries around the world, you will find required travel documents and immunizations. Follow the link to the Background Notes for detailed information about the region you want to visit, including history, government, economy, religion, political conditions, travel, and business information.

Travel Spots
www.travelspots.com

Click on a country name for detailed information including language, weather, maps, currency, local transportation and more. Includes fun things to do such as looking through cybercams at different areas. It also has travel puzzles and email postcards.

I Picture
www.ipicture.net

This comprehensive travel site lets you access pictures of your desired destination as well as link to websites for anything travel related. A "yellow pages" for travel websites, this is a good website to surf if you are not sure where you want to go.

U.S. Customs
www.customs.ustreas.gov/travel/travel.htm

This is another must-see site for information on Customs regulations and procedures that apply to travelers entering or exiting the United States. Their brochure, *Know Before You Go*, is an excellent resource.

On The Road
www.ontheroad.com

Mainly a domestic travel site, it also covers a few international destinations. You will learn about where to eat, what to see, and what events are going on in cities you are traveling to. Worth taking a look at to see if it can help you out with your research.

Embassy World
www.embassyworld.com

You can find the address and other information about the United States Embassy in the country in which you are traveling to or interested in.

Travelocity
www.travelocity.com

Any type of travel and all aspects of your trip can be researched on this site. There are tour ideas as well as information on how to book your own trip and obtaining the guides for your destination.

Arthur Frommer
www.frommers.com

This site will give you information on just about anything concerning travel and destinations. It has articles and travel tips available, as well as all Frommer publications. You can also email with specific questions.

Fodor's
www.fodors.com

This is one more site to check out when you are researching. They include quite a bit of travel information on destinations and up to date articles that you will be interested in viewing. They have links to several different websites that will be useful to your research.

Choosing Safe Transportation

Air

Air Safe
www.airsafe.com

For no-nonsense information on safety issues of air transportation, this is a must-see site. You will find statistics of air fatalities, accident reports, and service problems, and articles including air rage, how to deal with turbulence, and tips on how to care for children. They even provide information on what airlines and types of aircraft offer the best rides.

Sky-Guide
www.sky-guide.com

Sky-Guide is a subscriber site; for a nominal fee per year you can access flight schedules and information including departures, arrivals, and connecting flights. Operated by American Express, this is a great site for the businesswoman on the go.

Aircraft Disinsection Requirements
www.ostpxweb.dot.gov/policy/safey/disin.htm

This site will allow you to know which airlines and what countries require spraying of insecticides inside the cabin of the airplane. This will especially be useful if you have any problems with asthma or other breathing problems. You can also access the Centers for Disease Control for disinsection information at *www.cdc.gov*. (Follow links to *Travelers Health.*)

Official Airline Guide
www.oag.com

Frequent flyers have relied on the OAG flight guides for years. OAG is the one of the world's leading independent providers of essential travel information. Their database is used by travel agents, corporations, and airlines throughout the world, and provides customized timetables, flight schedules, and related data. Their pocket flight guide, available by subscription, is a must for business travelers. For example, if your flight is delayed, you can quickly access other flight schedules between your departure and arrival cities including the type of aircraft, food service, and number of stops. You can also access airport information such as locations of business centers, ATMs, etc.

United States Department of Transportation
www.dot.gov/airconsumer

This site is full of information and articles concerning air travel. If you go to the DOT home page you will find information on all forms of transportation.

International Airline Passengers Association
www.iapa.com

This is a membership traveler's association serving the frequent business traveler and is primarily geared towards the airline transportation industry. There are three tiers of membership, providing different benefits. You will be able to access what each airport offers in the way of clubs and amenities.

Rental Cars

Association for Safe International Road Travel
www.asirt.org

A great site if you are planning to drive or ride in a taxi or bus while in a foreign country. ASIRT is a non-profit organization that promotes road travel safety Their Road Travel Reports provide information about road conditions, driver behavior, vehicle maintenance, and the most dangerous roads in countries throughout the world. They have news for business travelers as well as tourists. They have a membership for businesspeople who travel often to foreign countries. This membership provides up-to-date statistics and information tailored to road travel in the destination country.

Rental Car Guide—www.rentalcarguide.com
Rental Cars—www.rentalcars.com

Both of these sites provide lists of car rental agencies serving airports in the U.S. and around the world. For example, click on London and you can find out what agencies serve Heathrow airport. They both have several pages on frequently asked questions about rental cars and some tips to go along with this information.

Smart Motorist
www.smartmotorist.com

This is a must-see site for motorists. It has a list of comprehensive articles covering everything from how to adjust your mirrors to what to do if you hit a deer. Dealing with fatigue and preventing car-jackings are just some of the health and safety topics that will assist you in your travel planning. Their advice comes from a variety of experts around the country.

Subway

> **Subway**
> www.metropla.net/

This is a great site for subway users. You can follow the links to subways systems around the world; for example, click on *euroMetro*, click on Paris, and you will find a detailed, colored map of the metro system in Paris. This site can be helpful in creating itineraries and making appointments. It also allows you to enter your departure location and destination, then it calculates the time it will take for you to get there.

Bus and Rail

> **Budget Travel**—www.budgettravel.com/eurobus.htm
> www.budgettravel.com/eurorail.htm

These sites provide links and information for rail and bus companies throughout Europe, including the websites for the bus systems of each individual country in eastern and western Europe. Be sure to research the company before booking with them.

> **Greyhound**
> www.greyhound.com

You can access bus fares and schedules around the U.S on this site as well as connection information with airlines and trains. Greyhound also offers tours and great student rates.

Accommodations

Hostels
www.hostels.com

This comprehensive site tells you all about hostels and what to expect when you arrive. You can navigate with ease through the site to find a directory of hostels in regions around the world. They give you phone numbers and addresses of all hostels as well as their email and website if available. You can access their message boards for discussions related to budget travel. Be sure to check out their *Hostelling 101* for answers to frequently asked questions about staying in hostels. This is a must-see site for budget travel planners.

Bed and Breakfast
www.bedandbreakfast.com

This Bed and Breakfast finder provides information on over 25,000 B&Bs and inns around the world. Follow the link to their map search to find accommodations in specific areas; for example, follow the map link to Denmark to find a list of 10 B&Bs in Copenhagen. You can also search by topics such as amenities and special deals.

Places to Stay
www.placestostay.com

This site is very user friendly and has an international directory of hotels, hostels, and bed and breakfasts. You will find rates as well as the area of the city in which the accommodations are located. They provide the web address and a brief description.

Accommodation Search Engine
www.ase.net

This site allows you to search the Web for accommodations exclusively in any country you choose. You can browse and review over 140,000 accommodation web pages from all over the world. Their search engine allows you to search by preferences such as rate, amenities, and facility requirements.

Hotel Guide
www.hotelguide.com

This hotel search site will allow you to enter any city worldwide and find a list of hotels, including rates in U.S. dollars. For example, enter Mexico City and you will receive a list of hotels with symbols showing whether they have pictures, website, and email addresses. We also like the world clock on the the homepage of this site.

All Hotels
www.all-hotels.com

You will find discounted rates and lots of travel information on this site. It is a "free membership" site so you will need to sign up to go into certain areas.

Global Assignment Americans Abroad
www.globalassignment.com

If you are concerned about how to protect yourself from travel risks such as the lack of cleanliness in some hotels, this site is for you. It has revolving articles about issues that face travelers. You can read current articles or access its archives for information such as how room attendants cut corners on cleaning rooms and how you can protect yourself against it.

Cruises

Cruise Lines International Association
www.cruising.org

This organization has strict guidelines for their members and provides great resources for cruise planning.

Concierge
www.concierge.com

This site, featuring *Conde Nast Traveler*, provides resources on choosing cruises and has sections on tipping and cruise disputes. Follow the link to *Cruise Guide*.

Cruise Reviews
www.cruiseopinion.com *and* www.cruisecritic.com

These websites are great resources for reviews by cruise passengers. You can search their databases for reviews for specific cruise lines.

Great Tools for the Traveling Woman

Executive Planet
www.executiveplanet.com/community

Your guide to international business etiquette and culture, this is a great place to learn about protocol in the country of your interest. You may find out that it is not advisable to give a business contact a gift in China, or that in the Philippines skirts should be knee-length while necklines should remain conservative. Find out where women should avoid wearing pants or pantsuits. This is an especially useful website for businesswomen and one of our favorite sites for the international traveler.

Kropla
www.kropla.com

Steve Kropla has the latest information on electrical and phone access abroad. The site provides a list of electrical travel accessories you can and cannot use in the country you are traveling to. It also gives the international dialing codes as well as what type of television programming is offered by different countries. Steve includes easy-to-understand diagrams showing different plug types and even using electronic equipment such as modem hook-ups. If you want to know if your curling iron will work in Singapore, check out this site before you go.

Travelers Aid
www.travelersaid.com

Traveler's Aid International's member agencies serve individuals and families in crisis due to homelessness, mobility, or other disruptive circumstances. They are found at many airports around the world as well as some bus and train stations. We accessed the Travelers Aid office at Chicago O'Hare International Airport where volunteers assisted travelers with everything from band-aids to directions. Access their website for locations at your travel destination or en route.

Weather Channel
www.weather.com

This is one of many weather sites that you can access. You can find out the weather and related information that will be a great help in planning what to pack and what type of clothing to take on your trip.

Council Travel
www.counciltravel.com

This site for traveling students has an abundance of information. Students can order rail passes at a discount and get an ID card that will allow discounts at different places worldwide. It also has a page for students to access information on different study programs.

Safe Within
www.safewithin.com

This is a comprehensive site on safety from home to travel, from children to seniors. You will find tips on how to make your home and your travels safe.

World Room
www.worldroom.com

Although based in Asia, this site is full of travel news and information for the business traveler. Click on their link to *Women's World,* where you will find articles for the traveling woman, great tips, and links to other women's travel sites. It provides free email as well as links to airlines and hotels. We also love the design of this site: interesting, full of information, yet easy to navigate.

Health

Medicine Planet
www.medicineplanet.com

We love this site for information on travel health, especially the in-depth advice for traveling women. To access parts of this site you will need to become a member, although membership is free. They have a comprehensive view of the country on which you would like information, from its population to addresses of important offices. It is, however, mainly a site focused on how to stay healthy while on your trip. They also offer a link to a service that will translate your medications into the language of the country you are visiting, which may be helpful if you run out or lose yours.

World Health Organization
www.who.int/

For information about health issues in countries around the world, this organization can provide up-to-date information that may be critical for you to know before traveling. WHO is a directing and coordinating authority on health work and provides information on this website that can assist you in planning your travel. When you access the site, you will find links to information such as disease outbreaks in countries around the world. To access information about a specific country, go to "WHO regional and other offices." This will lead you to a page with links for the country you are interested in.

Travel Health Online
www.tripprep.com

You will find at this site a list of all health and disease problems for any country. It warns you of problems and outbreaks and tells you how to keep yourself safe. It gives you a list of travel medicine providers and keeps you up to date on traveler information.

Centers for Disease Control and Prevention
www.cdc.gov

Here, you will be able to determine what diseases or outbreaks are occurring around the world. It has an abundance of articles and information for you to access, including a list of immunizations that may be required before traveling. For example, follow the link to *Traveler's Health*, click on Central Africa, and you will find comprehensive information about the region: disease outbreaks, vaccines for prevention and treatment of diseases, and travel tips for staying healthy while visiting this area. A must-see site for travelers going to Third World countries. You can also follow the link to *Cruise Ships* for "Sanitation and Inspections of International Cruise Ships" reports and *Air Travel* for disinfection information.

Travel Health Online
www.tripprep.com/index.html

On this site you will find a variety of travel health issues listed in an easy-to-find chart. It describes what the issue or illness is and then gives you ideas and precautions to help you through the process.

> **International Association for Medication Assistance to Travellers**—www.sentex.net/~iamat

Worth checking out, this is a free membership site from a non-profit foundation and is designed to make available to travelers around the world competent medical care by Western-trained doctors who speak English. Members receive quite a few benefits.

Travelers Insurance

There are many different options when choosing travel insurance: baggage insurance, trip interruption insurance, and life and medical insurance. The following websites give you several choices and allow you to pick the best fit for your needs.

> **World Travel Center**
> www.worldtravelcenter.com

> **Council Travel**
> www.counciltravel.com/travelinsurance

> **Global Travel Insurance**
> www.globaltravelinsurance.com

Other Great Sites for the Traveling Woman

> **The Traveling Woman**
> www.thetravelingwoman.net *or* www.travelingsafe.com

This is our site, designed to share resources to encourage safe and healthy travel for women. Our company TravelingSafe.com, was formed to educate women on the concepts that **an edu-cated traveler is a safer traveler** and that personal health and safety habits should become a lifestyle. We offer a weekly tip and links to other great websites focused on women who travel.

iShopAroundTheWorld
www.ishoparoundtheworld.com

Although not a site designed exclusively for women only, we love to shop, and this is a great resource website for information about shopping and traveling around the world. Based on their travel guidebooks, *Treasures and Pleasures of...Best of the Best*, veteran travelers Ron and Caryl Krannich offer a global shopping directory, community forum, and travel tips. Love shopping for antiques? Click on this link to find names of shops and recommendations in countries from A-Z.

Passenger Rights
www.passengerrights.com

A site where you can be heard and maybe, just maybe, you will hear back from someone. You will be able to air your grievances on this site, and they will forward them on to the proper departments. Who knows what will happen.

Currency & Credit Cards

Oanda
www.oanda.com

This is a currency rate converter site; however, it does do more than conversions. You can discuss with others the current conversion rates and why they fluctuate. If you go into *oanda.com/convert/cheatsheet* you can print out a full conversion chart.

Currency-to-go
www.currency-to-go.com

Step off the plane with foreign currency in hand for taxis, tips, and snacks. Have it delivered right to your door or any local Chase Bank branch the next business day. Order up to $1,000 in any combination of foreign currency, foreign currency travelers checks, and U.S. dollar travelers checks. Free home delivery when your total order is $500 or more.

Catalogs

Magellans
www.magellans.com

This shopping site has all the travel paraphernalia you would ever need. You can order a free catalog online or call toll free to order their catalog (domestic phone number 800-962-4943 and international 805-568-5400). We love their products designed to make traveling safer and easier.

Travel Smith
www.travelsmith.com

This is also a great travel-related shopping site, offering a complete line of travel clothes that will no doubt fit all your needs. Check this site out if you need wrinkle-free clothing.

About the Authors

Veteran travelers, **Catherine Comer** and **Lavon Swaim** hold degrees in tourism management and own TravelingSafe.com, a company focused on providing travel safety information.

Catherine's travel experience began over fifteen years ago when she accompanied her husband as he worked internationally and throughout the U.S. On her own, she explored cities such as Madrid, Sydney, and London, gaining experience in how to enjoy travel with safety in mind. With a background in marketing, Catherine decided to focus on a career in the tourism industry. She has traveled to destinations around the world and led a government delegation for Oregon's participation in the 1999 International Travel Expo in South Korea. Her career has included forming a visitor association for Oregon's fourth largest city where she developed a tourism marketing strategy and designed and produced marketing brochures. She was named Livable Oregon's 1995 Main Street Manager of the Year for her work in developing a downtown revitalization and marketing program.

Lavon has been a travel planner for international groups and a tour guide for senior citizen groups traveling throughout the U.S. Her experience began 15 years ago when she traveled on her own from the West Coast to New York. Her love of travel led her to a career in the tourism industry. While traveling to South America to participate in a mission outreach, she was stranded overnight in an Argentine airport, where she had to sleep on the floor. This prompted her to study travel safety issues for women. Her experience has enabled her to teach women travelers how to develop good travel safety habits. Lavon has also been a resort sales manager and a visitor center representative.

Catherine and Lavon have given numerous presentations and workshops in a variety of venues. As professional women who have traveled for both business and leisure, they represent the target audience for *THE TRAVELING WOMAN*. "We are women who love to travel and believe that whether a woman is traveling on her own, with a spouse or partner, or in a group, she should know and practice personal safety habits as a lifestyle."

Catherine and Lavon can be reached at
email@TheTravelingWoman.net or 503-618-0241

Index

The Click and Easy™ Online Resource Centers —

Books, videos, software, training materials, articles, and advice for travelers, job seekers, employers, HR professionals, schools, and libraries.

Visit us online for all your travel and career needs. Includes a comprehensive travel bookstore, shopping carts, an international travel-shopping center, and several downloadable catalogs in PDF format:

www.ImpactPublications.com
(bookstores and Impact Publications)

www.iShopAroundTheWorld.com
(unique international travel-shopping center)

www.ContentForTravel.com
(syndicated travel content for travelers
and travel professionals)

www.WinningTheJob.com
(career articles, advice, and bookstore)

www.ContentForCareers.com
(syndicated career content for job seekers,
employees, and Intranets)

www.GreenToGray.com
www.BlueToGray.com
(military transition databases and content)